A Down-to-Earth Approach to Being a Nurse Educator

Victoria Schoolcraft, R.N., Ph.D., is Professor and Associate Dean for the Undergraduate Program at Barry University School of Nursing, Miami Shores, Florida. She was formerly Associate Professor and Assistant Director for the Baccalaureate Program at the University of Oklahoma College of Nursing. She received her B.S.N. from the University of Oklahoma; an M.S.N. from the University of Texas School of Nursing at Austin; and her Ph.D. in higher education administration from the University of Oklahoma College of Education. She is a member of the Florida Nurses Association/American Nurses Association, Sigma Theta Tau, and Phi Delta Kappa.

Dr. Schoolcraft wrote *A Nuts-and-Bolts Approach to Teaching Nursing* (Springer, 1989), which was Volume 11 in the Springer Series on the Teaching of Nursing. Dr. Schoolcraft was the editor and principal author for *Nursing in the Community* (Wiley, 1984). She is interested in all aspects of education and socialization of nursing educators. Her dissertation and continuing research interests concern the phenomenon of mentorship.

Dr. Schoolcraft has been an educator for 20 years. Although she has been an administrator of nursing education for 13 of those years, she has continued to be active in teaching undergraduate and graduate nursing students.

A Down-to-Earth Approach to Being a Nurse Educator

VICTORIA SCHOOLCRAFT, RN, PhD

SPRINGER PUBLISHING COMPANY • NEW YORK

Springer Publishing Company, Inc.
536 Broadway
New York, NY 10012

94 95 96 97 98 / 5 4 3 2 1

Library of Congress Cataloging-in-Publication Data

Schoolcraft, Victoria.
    A down-to-earth approach to being a nurse educator / Victoria Schoolcraft.
        p.   cm. — (Springer series on the teaching of nursing ; v. 16)
    Includes bibliographical references and index.
    ISBN 0−8261−8130−9
    1. Nursing schools—Faculty.   2. Nursing—Vocational guidance.
I. Title.   II. Series.
    [DNLM: 1. Faculty, Nursing.   2. Vocational Guidance.   W1 SP685SG
v. 16 1994 / WY 19 S3715d 1994]
RT90.S298   1994
610.73'071'1—dc20
DNLM/DLC
for Library of Congress   93-34776
                                                                               CIP

Printed in the United States of America

To one of my first and always
one of my best mentors

Martha Compton Primeaux

and

To one of my first and always
one of my best mentees

Caryn Stoermer Hess

Contents

Preface

This book is intended as a practical resource for new nurse faculty members beginning their careers in academia. From landing a teaching job to honing communication, writing, and research skills, and finding your place as a member of a scholarly community, I have tried to offer "down-to-earth" advice to new faculty members seeking to develop and grow in their careers. I hope more experienced faculty members will be able to find useful information here as well, for making their careers even more dynamic.

I saw this book as a necessary companion to my earlier book, *A Nuts and Bolts Approach to Teaching Nursing*, which is a guide to the actual teaching itself. Finishing this second book was like finishing my autobiography—describing what I had learned in a life spent in the teaching of nursing.

When I first submitted my proposal for this book to Dr. Rita Wieczorek and Springer Publishing Company, I was very enthusiastic and eager to get started. *Nuts and Bolts* had been a joy to write. In fact, it practically wrote itself. However, some personal events intervened to slow down my writing progress, and when I was able to work on the book again, I found it difficult to construct each chapter. Before long, I had skeletons of each one, but very little meat on those bones. I had to make myself work on this book. Each day as I sat down at my computer, I struggled with trying to flesh out each chapter with meaning. Many times I shut down the computer with a sense that all I had done was to rearrange the words.

After months of dreading each encounter with this project, I suddenly had a flash of insight. I was working again on the chapter about becoming part of the organization. I started writing about how I had felt as a new faculty member in my current position. For the first time, I realized that my feelings had been what was missing. When I started using my own experiences and feelings to help illustrate points, the writing flowed more easily and the book really began to take shape. Thus, this book has a different, more personal flavor than *Nuts and Bolts*. But I hope that new faculty members will find it equally useful in establishing the foundations of a flourishing career.

VICTORIA SCHOOLCRAFT
North Miami, FL

Acknowledgments

If this is a helpful book, I owe its helpfulness to a lot of wise and helpful people I have had contact with in my personal and my professional lives. To start with the personal, I thank my parents, Barbara and RA. They believed in me all my life. When I graduated from high school, my dad was recently retired from the Air Force. He was struggling with a new civilian career and had a tight income, considering there were five children in the family. Many of my friends were going on to business and technical schools, but my folks were determined that I should go to college. While I was an undergraduate, they helped me to succeed in every way possible. I even changed my major several times, which extended my schooling. Once someone asked me if my parents had especially wanted me to become a nurse. I said, "No, they wanted me to become a graduate." That was fact, but in truth, they wanted me to be successful and happy, so they gave me as much as they could (and sometimes more) to help while I was in school. There's hardly any way to properly thank your parents for doing what they do just because they're your parents. The way I have tried to thank mine is to be successful and happy and to let them know that I appreciate the good start they gave me on this journey. Thanks Mom and Dad.

I have been blessed with a wonderful set of siblings, two brothers and two sisters who have been my friends as well. Bob, Mike, Mary Chloe, and San have brought so much joy to my life. I always look forward to our times together and treasure the memories of times past. Two of them have married wonderful people to bring into our family. Suzie is married to Bob. She has helped me many times in ways in-laws aren't often given credit for. John

Saunders married Mary Chloe and has become my friend as well as my brother-in-law. My sister San died unexpectedly while this book was in production, but she has always been and will always be part of anything I do.

Most of my closest friends are nurses and many are nurse educators as well. I have shared so much with them that weaves in and out of my personal and professional endeavors. I will risk naming some, hoping those who don't get named will be placated with bribes later. Some of these friends and helpers include: Sr. Peggy Albert, Tom Allen, Rosemarie Apple, Dr. Judith Balcerski, Dr. Quilla Bell-Turner, Dr. Melba Cather, Clare Delaney, Dr. Patricia Dolphin, Caryn Stoermer Hess, Sheila Hopkins, Dr. Sharol Jacobson, Louise McCormick, Evelyn McKennon, Linda Perkel, Martha Primeaux, Dr. Gloria Smith, Loretta Thompson, and Keith Tyler.

As far as those wise helpers in my professional life, most of the above have contributed to some extent. However, I should say that the people who had the most impact on my professional development and my own experience of learning how to be a faculty member have been: Dr. Judith Balcerski, my current dean at Barry University; Dr. Sharol Jacobson, Director of Research at the University of Oklahoma College of Nursing (OUCN) who served on my dissertation committee; Martha Primeaux, former Assistant Dean and Director of the Baccalaureate Program at OUCN when I worked there; and Dr. Gloria Smith who was the dean at OUCN for the majority of the time I taught there. These fine academicians provided rich environments for growth, sent me to professional meetings, and praised my accomplishments.

There are two other creatures I want to thank for their companionship and special support during the writing of this book. However, they'll never read their names in print. They are my two cats, Tegan and Sooner. They frequently supervise my work from the top of my computer monitor or nap with their heads on the corner of my keyboard.

Finally, I want to thank Dr. Ursula Springer, Dr. Rita Wieczorek, Matt Fenton, and Ruth Chasek at Springer Publishing Company for the confidence and support that gave me the opportunity to work on this book.

Author's Note

Throughout this book, the term "university" will be used to designate the parent institution; "school" will be used for the academic unit for nursing; and "dean" will be used to designate the chief administrator in the school.

ONE

Finding and Getting a Faculty Position

•••••••••••••••••••••••••••••••

$There$ are many ways to accomplish the goal expressed in the title of this chapter. I plan to discuss not only how you identify positions for which you qualify, but also how to make a positive impression on those who interview you. Due to the nature of my career, I've interviewed many prospective faculty members. However, I haven't changed positions frequently myself. Therefore, my perspective is that of the person looking for a new faculty member, rather than that of the person searching for a position.

PURPOSES

This chapter will help you to:

- identify potential positions that you might choose;
- make appropriate contacts in investigating a prospective position;
- prepare a professional curriculum vitae; and
- present yourself well in the interview.

LOOKING FOR A POSITION

Unless you have a spectacular reputation or some special attributes, you will probably have to go looking for a position. Faculty positions are sometimes advertised in regular newspapers, especially in large metropolitan areas. However, budgets for the search process are no less constrained than others, so people are going to advertise where they will get "more bang for their bucks." That means you're more likely to find what you want in professional publications.

The *Chronicle of Higher Education* is an excellent resource. Most colleges advertise there for faculty searches. Other journals that reach a general audience may carry position descriptions, especially if the people they are looking for are hard to find. For example, *Nursing and Health Care* and *Nursing Outlook* are frequent advertising outlets because of the nature of their readership. So are the *Journal of Nursing Education* and *Nurse Educator*. In addition, you will want to look in any specialty journals for the given field in which you can teach.

Tell people you know that you are interested in a particular kind of position. They may know of appropriate positions, or be more likely to pay attention to such notices if they know what you're interested in. Look at the job boards available at the school where you are a student or an instructor. If you are moving to or have just relocated to a new area, send letters to schools there and enclose your curriculum vitae. They may be searching for someone, but you might have missed their notices. Even if these schools have no openings, they will usually file your C.V. for future reference.

Frequently, people are looking for prospective faculty members at regional, state, or national meetings. Often there is a particular bulletin board with such notices posted. If the school has a booth in the exhibit area, you can inquire about openings.

MAKING APPLICATION

The position notice will usually specify what you should do to apply. Initially, this will usually include, submission of a cover letter describing yourself and your abilities, accompanied by your curriculum vitae. Your letter should include the following:

- how you found out about the opening;
- why you are looking for a position;
- terms of your availability for the position;

- summary of your education;
- summary of your experience as a nurse and as a teacher; and
- your availability for the interview process.

The letter should be succinct and look professional. A sample cover letter is shown in Table 1.1.

CURRICULUM VITAE

You should follow a standard format for your curriculum vitae (C.V.). If you are already on a faculty, your school may have a preferred format for you to follow. A sample format is shown in the Appendix.

Your C.V. is a summary of your professional life. You should have a complete one, but for many purposes, you may modify it to show your activities over the most recent three to five years. The person or group requesting your C.V. may specify its scope in terms of time. For most C.V. purposes, you will always include the following:

- current address and telephone;
- all your education, degrees, and dates;
- all licensure information;
- all your professional positions, locations, and dates;
- all your publications; and
- all your completed research and research in progress.

The remaining areas will probably reflect only your recent activities:

- continuing education taught;
- continuing education attended;
- membership in professional organizations, including offices and committees;
- professional meetings attended and presentations made;
- community service; and
- consultation.

Table 1.1

Cover Letter

Mary C. Lowe, R.N., M.S.N.
5050 Deely Road
Kansas City, MO 64100
January 19, 1992

Muriel Morris, R.N., Ph.D.
Associate Professor
Chair, Search Committee
College of Nursing
Walker University
Miami Groves, FL 33130

Dear Dr. Morris:

I would like to apply for the position of instructor in pediatric nursing, which I saw advertised in the *Chronicle of Higher Education*. I am currently on the faculty at the School of Nursing at Henderson University in Kansas City, MO, and will be moving to Florida to enter the doctoral program at Walker University.

My teaching responsibilities have included the preparation and presentation of lectures, clinical supervision of undergraduate students, and academic advisement. In addition, I have served on the College of Nursing Curriculum Committee for the least year and a half. I have also served as a consulting committee member in supervising two MSN students who were working on theses relating to the care of children with cancer.

My primary clinical interest is in working with children who have cancer and with their families. However, I have maintained my clinical skills and still work well in a general pediatric setting.

If you choose to interview me for this position, I can come to Miami Groves almost any time except early May, when our semester will be ending. Due to my teaching schedule, an interview on a Thursday or Friday would be most convenient for me.

My direct superior is Dr. Linda Campbell, the Associate Dean for Undergraduate Programs at the College of Nursing. She is aware that I am inquiring about this position, and has stated that she is more than willing to furnish a written and/or a telephone reference for me. Additional references will be furnished at your request.

Thank you for considering my application. I will look forward to hearing from you. I can be reached at 1−816−555−3937 during the day and at 1−816−555−5566 in the evening.

Sincerely,
Mary C. Lowe, R.N., M.S.N.

INTERVIEWING

There are two steps in interviewing: preparing for it, and actually doing it. The better prepared you are, the more comfortable you will feel in the interview, and the better you will do.

PREPARATION

Get as much information as you can about the school and the university. Once an interview date is set, ask for a university catalog and any other information that can easily be sent. The history of the institution is usually given in a thumbnail sketch. From this you can get a picture of how the university grew and what affiliations are relevant. For example, you can learn whether it is private or public; if it has a connection to a particular religious group; if it is noted for particular academic units; or if it serves in some special way as a part of the community.

Catalogs also list the degrees offered by the institution and the schools that comprise it. In this way you can get an idea of the resources available and the diversity of the faculty and student body.

Read all the information you can get about the school of nursing. Some of the things that you should look for are listed below:

- administrative structure of the school;
- curriculum framework;
- date of last NLN site visit;
- names of the dean and other administrators;
- names of the search committee members and description of their roles, if available;
- NLN accreditation status;
- numbers of enrolled students and annual graduates;
- organizational structures of the school and university;
- philosophies and mission statements of the school and the university, and
- programs, options, and majors offered within the school.

If you know anyone who has attended, graduated from, taught at, or even visited the school or university, talk with them to get an idea of what it is like. If you know people in the area local to the university, contact them for their knowledge about it. If you live near the university but have never been there, take a walk or drive around the campus. Walking is better, because you get more of the "feel" of the place than you can by driving around.

If you live far from the area, look it up on a map to get an idea of its proximity to local resources. If you can arrive early for the interview, go to the campus ahead of time to walk around and investigate.

As you go through your reading material and look the campus over, make notes about things you want to clarify. Write down your questions about the school, the university, and the local area. Write down your questions about the specific position you are interviewing for.

You should also make notes about anything about yourself that you particularly want to emphasize. You might want to take some documentation with you to indicate your strengths, and may be asked to bring things with you for the search committee's perusal. For example, if you put together a study packet for an independent study course, you might want to show that packet to the search committee to demonstrate your abilities in doing such things. If you have any publications or research reports, you may want to plan on taking them with you, but these should probably be shared only if you are requested to do so.

THE INTERVIEW

Request a schedule of the activities to be involved in your interview process. You may be interviewed by a committee as well as by some additional individuals, and you will feel more prepared if you know in advance to whom you will be talking. At the minimum, interviewers usually include a search committee, the course coordinator with whom you'd be working most closely, and the dean or associate dean.

I can't think of any recent occasion when a prospective faculty member appeared for an interview in inappropriate attire. However, I will still mention this as an important consideration. Dress in a professional manner. Don't wear too much jewelry, make-up, or cologne. Wear something in which you feel comfortable and which makes you look your best. Carry a notepad or briefcase, if you wish, but you should at least have something with which to take notes.

When you're introduced to people, take note of their names and titles, and write down this information as soon as possible. Look people in the eye when you talk with them. Remember to smile occasionally. After all, the people interviewing you are your colleagues in the discipline of nursing.

In most interview situations, there will be a certain amount of small talk while you're waiting for others to arrive, or while you're being escorted to the next place. Try to relax and be genuine when you chat about nursing or other interests during these interludes.

Some people have interview formats they follow in asking questions of candidates. This helps to ensure that each person interviewed has the opportunity to respond to the same things. Some of the things that might be asked about, even if the information is included in your C.V., include:

- your philosophy of nursing;
- your philosophy of teaching;
- a description of your teaching experiences;
- a description of your clinical experiences;
- your writing and research activities;
- your participation in professional organizations;
- your contributions to community service;
- your personal and professional goals;
- your reasons for being interested in the particular position for which you're interviewing; and
- any special qualifications related to the particular position.

If there are any gaps in your experience, or if you are aware of any deficiencies you might have in relation to the position for which you're interviewing, be prepared to address these problems and discuss how you will remedy them. It is often difficult for the employer to find a prospective faculty member who is exactly what they're looking for. Therefore, employers will have to choose among candidates with various combinations of strengths and weaknesses and decide which combination is the best fit. If you do your best to show how you can fit your prospective employer's needs, your chances of getting the position you want will be improved.

Usually the search committee and/or the course coordinator will describe what the particular position involves. They will also give you other information about teaching in the school and the other responsibilities you would have.

As I mentioned above, you should have questions of your own to bring up when appropriate. You should ask any questions you couldn't answer through your own research. This helps to show your preparedness and helps you to know more about what you're getting into. Make sure you clarify exactly what the position will require, as well as the support available for doing the job.

Generally, the administrator to whom you will report will give you information about the salary and benefits involved. Ask how the employer's salary structure compares to the American Association of Colleges of Nursing (AACN) statistics for similar schools. Clarify what other things might be expected of you as part of your contract, in addition to the obvious responsibilities of a teaching position. For example, you may be expected to serve on a certain number of committees, carry a particular advising load, attend certain events, and so on. Make sure you know when the position is available and when you would be expected to start work if it was offered to you.

You are very likely to feel somewhat nervous during the interview process, especially if you really want the position. The people interviewing you will know that this nervousness is normal. As a matter of fact, if you don't seem a little nervous you might come across as arrogant and uninterested. I'm not saying you should act nervous if you're not—just don't worry about showing a little anxiety. If your interviewers can't tolerate that, they probably wouldn't be very supportive to work with, either. Usually, once you start talking, you will start relaxing.

Some general things to try to keep in mind are:

- stay on the topic of discussion;
- don't give long rambling answers;
- give succinct but complete responses to questions;
- be specific about your own questions; and
- avoid getting off on tangents.

Another important issue that deserves emphasis is the way that you talk about other people. No matter how difficult previous colleagues have been to deal with, don't use your interview as a place to dump these feelings. Avoid negative and judgmental remarks about people you've worked with. Even if you are perfectly justified in your assessments, such comments may reflect more on you than on the people you're describing. Be as diplomatic as possible in describing the events leading up to your making a move if the reasons for your relocation are related to difficulties in dealing with others. The person or persons you had difficulty with in your previous position could be respected by, or even be friends with, someone who is interviewing you.

Before you leave the interview site, clarify, what additional information, if any, your prospective employers need from you before making their decision. If there is any additional material they intend to give you, clarify who will be sending it and when. Ask when you might be hearing about the outcome of their deliberations. If you will be reimbursed for any expenses you incurred in coming to the interview, clarify the procedure involved to arrange for this.

AFTER THE INTERVIEW

After the interview, send any additional information requested, and do so as quickly as possible. If you are being reimbursed for expenses, submit the necessary information and receipts in a timely manner. Review what you learned in the interview. Discuss your interview with a friend or colleague in order to assess your wishes to accept the position if it's offered to you.

You should be notified by telephone or in writing whether or not the position is being offered to you. Usually, this notification will include something about why you were or were not selected. If the position is not offered to you, you should accept this as graciously as possible. Write a letter to the administrator who interviewed you and send a copy to the chair of the search committee. Thank these people for their time and effort, and let them know of any interest in being considered again in the future. An example of such a letter is in Table 1.2.

If the position is offered to you, this will usually be done in a telephone call. You may already be certain that you want to accept with no further deliberation on your part. If you feel that way, say so. Clarify what is being offered and your responsibilities. You

Table 1.2

Letter in Response to Unoffered Position

Maribel Thurman, R.N., Ph.D.
Director
Department of Nursing
Littlefield College
Littlefield, SD 57501

Dear Dr. Thurman:

Thank you for notifying me about the instructor position for which I applied. I understand that a more experienced faculty member was selected.

Thank you very much for considering me for the position. I enjoyed meeting you and the other faculty members involved. Please keep me in mind should another position become available.

Sincerely,

Benjamin Kelley, R.N., M.S.N.

cc: Dr. Charlotte Murphy
      Chair, Search Committee

may be asked to write a letter of intent or sign a form stating your intent to accept the position while your contract is prepared. You should respond to this request immediately.

If the position is offered and you have not yet decided if you want it, ask for a reasonable amount of time, usually a few days, to think it over. If you are a young and inexperienced faculty member and you know there have been several applicants for the position, you can't afford to spend too much time thinking about accepting or not accepting the position. If you decide to decline the offer, telephone the person who offered it as soon as possible. Follow up with a gracious letter. An example of such a letter is in Table 1.3.

Table 1.3

Letter Declining a Position

Maribel Thurman, R.N., Ph.D.
Director
Department of Nursing
Littlefield College
Littlefield, SD 57501

Dear Dr. Thurman:

Thank you for offering me the instructor position for which I applied. As I told you on the telephone, I was offered a similar position nearer to where I now live. I have decided it would be a better choice for me at this time to not move so far away.

Thank you very much for considering me for the position. I enjoyed meeting you and the other faculty members involved.

Sincerely,

Benjamin Kelley, R.N., M.S.N.

CONCLUSION

When you are a neophyte in academia, your choices of positions may be more limited than those you may eventually enjoy. However, there will still be many opportunities worth investigating. As with any job search, the better prepared you are, the more effectively your time will be spent. Whether or not you are offered a position you desire, you should end your association with the people who interviewed you on a positive note.

·············TWO·············

Orienting to the Position and Place

•••••••••••••••••••••••••••••••

Newcomers to organizations have certain character-
istic responses to unfamiliar settings. The novice's initial experiences have an impact on her or his eventual integration and
socialization into the organization. When new faculty members
understand these events and appreciate the process of socialization, they can have a smoother transition as they become part of a
faculty group.

PURPOSES

This chapter will help you to:

- clarify your expectations and the expectations of others as
  you become part of an organization;
- identify what is required in the position you are taking;
- identify important information about the school and the
  university; and
- get organized to have an effective entry experience.

SOCIALIZATION

Socialization is the process by which individuals learn the knowledge and skills which will help them to become effective members

of a group. During socialization a person learns the norms and values appropriate to their new role. Even if you are already an experienced faculty member, you will go through this process if you take on a new role or move into a different group. Louis (1980) has identified three stages of socialization:

1.   Anticipatory socialization: Outsiders develop expectations about their new role and about the organization, some of which may be unrealistic.

2.   Encounter: Outsiders become newcomers and their expectations are tested; differences between expectations and reality may lead to "reality shock."

3.   Adaptation: Newcomers become insiders after proving themselves, gain access to more information, and are sought out for advice.

DEVELOPING EXPECTATIONS

We can expect that in any encounter between prospective faculty members and potential employers, those on each side will be putting forward their best appearance. You will want to show a search committee or dean who might hire you all your strengths and best abilities and downplay any weaknesses. By the same token, the search committee and dean will present you with the most positive view they can of their organization. This is a normal part of the hiring process, but it can lead to incorrect expectations of one participant on the part of the other.

You should try to be as direct as you can about your concerns and questions. You will develop more accurate expectations if the preview of your job is as realistic as possible. The less you check out when you're interviewing and after you are hired, the more room there will be for unrealistic expectations.

Once you have accepted a position, you must start learning about it. You need to be realistic about your preconceptions as you develop them. However, since many expectations are developed unconsciously, the only way you become aware of them is when they are suddenly proven wrong. For example, you may have the unspoken expectation that you will have release time to work on your research. If this is a strong assumption, you may not even ask about it at the interview. However, once you arrive, you may find out that your teaching, advising, and meeting schedule is much too heavy to allow time for your research activities.

Furthermore, once you have accepted the position, you may start developing even more assumptions which you need to test. Some issues about which people develop expectations are:

- access to resources;
- advisee load;
- appropriate attire;
- assistance for novice teachers;
- availability of a mentor or guide;
- committee activities and responsibilities;
- employee benefits;
- involvement in crucial planning and decisions;
- office size and amenities;
- opportunities for advancement;
- other opportunities, such as teaching different levels of students;
- professional leave time;
- relationships with other schools within the university;
- release time for research;
- secretarial or similar support;
- support services within the university; and
- teaching responsibilities.

Although you may touch on some of these questions while considering a position, they may seem less important to you before you have actually accepted a position. While you are preparing to enter your new position, you should find out about the issues mentioned above, as well as others you might think of as you peruse this list. This will minimize the effects of "reality shock" when you actually arrive to assume your new role.

TESTING EXPECTATIONS

As a newcomer, you will begin to test the expectations you have developed. You will also realize that even with your intent to make these expectations conscious, conflict will still be apparent when an unconscious assumption is tested.

Most institutions have some kind of orientation available for faculty members. The nature and extent of this orientation varies widely from as little as half a day to as much as a year-long program of regular activities for new faculty members. Time and money constraints, and not need, often determine the length and breadth of such activities. Therefore, do not assume that the orientation plan at your institution is necessarily that which is most useful. You may find that you need to take an active role in finding out what you need to know, because no one else may have the time to do this with you.

In addition to the expectations enumerated earlier, as you move toward becoming an insider you will want to test other aspects of the system. Some of the things to look for include:

- attention given by faculty and administrators to following policies;
- degree of faculty involvement in decision making;
- displays of respect, or lack of respect, among faculty;
- indicators of how much teaching is valued;
- moods and behaviors of co-workers;
- openness to change;
- overt and covert indicators of faculty members' attitudes toward students;
- politics within and outside the school; and
- which faculty members hold places of influence, and who has influence upon whom.

SENSE MAKING

Several years ago, I ran across a fascinating article by Meryl Reis Louis (1980) which discusses the concept of "surprise and sense making" in relation to newcomers entering organizations. Human beings tend to try to make sense of new experiences or frame them in some way to make them understandable. Fundamentally, this concept involves the following process:

1. Newcomers give meaning to their new experiences based on their past experiences, and this may lead to inappropriate or dysfunctional interpretations;

2. Newcomers may attribute permanence to temporary situations, or vice versa;

3 Newcomers may see themselves as the source or cause of events, when external factors are responsible; and

4. Newcomers may overpersonalize their attributions of meaning to unexpected events.

Obviously this process can describe almost any new experience. Stop and think for a moment as you look back over those descriptors and apply them to some new experience you have had recently. An example of this process in action is given in Situation 2.1.

HELP FROM INSIDERS

A great disadvantage facing newcomers is that they do not know many colleagues well enough to ask for help in making sense of surprising events. As a newcomer, you need to identify some insiders, if they are not identified for you, who will help you to test reality when you are confronted with unexpected events. Identifying the right people may be difficult, since they are part of what is unfamiliar to you.

Some things to consider when you are looking for insiders to be your guides or mentors are that these people are:

- assured and confident of their own positions;
- available to help in the way you need help;
- aware and knowledgeable about what you need to know;
- capable of providing you with the kind of support you need;
- considerate and understanding of newcomers;
- respected by other faculty and recent newcomers; and
- unthreatened by you.

Louis (1980) suggests that insiders can help to test your perceptions and interpretations, and provide you with a different perspective of the events that concern you. They may have factual information that can help you understand a situation like the one described in Situation 2.1. For example, an insider might be well aware of the politics at play that bewilder you in the committee meeting. A helpful insider can give you information so that you

Situation 2.1

Surprise and Sense Making

Dora Nobles was a new faculty member who volunteered for the Grants and Awards Committee for the university. At her first meeting, she introduced herself to Paul Fielding, the chairperson. She told him she was a new faculty member and also new to teaching. He said, "OK. Sit over there." During the meeting, Fielding did not introduce her nor did he ask anyone else for introductions. Several times during the meeting, he allowed Dan Morton, another faculty member, to speak without being recognized. This faculty member elaborated at length about his concerns about a new policy for funding intramural research proposals. When Nobles tried to contribute to the discussion, Fielding interrupted her and said, "You should raise your hand so I can recognize you before you speak." Other members of the group were virtually silent, and no one was friendly to Nobles, although they often whispered comments to one another or passed each other notes. When the meeting concluded, Nobles asked Fielding when the next meeting would be held. He glanced at his watch and said, "Look, I'm in a hurry. I don't have time to nurse you along." With that he turned and walked off, leaving Nobles standing by herself.

Of course, there are many human responses Nobles might have to this encounter. She might have past experience recognizing that sometimes people are rude or act inappropriately through no fault of her own. If so, she may conclude that Fielding's behavior in the foregoing meeting was related to something to do with him, and perhaps had little to do with her. On the other hand, if she felt insecure, she might interpret Fielding's behavior as a response to her inexperience as a faculty member. She might feel that she was the one who was behaving incorrectly.

The truth of the situation was that Fielding was an assistant professor ready to apply for promotion to associate professor. Dan Morton was an influential member of the Rank and Promotion Committee. Other faculty members, realizing that Fielding was catering to Morton, decided to avoid getting caught in the middle. All the committee members besides Noble were operating out of their own needs for self-preservation, and were uninterested in being of service to a newcomer.

can avoid surprises and learn to understand the subtleties of the situation not easily accessible to a new person.

You must be aware of the insider's needs and motivations. This is one factor that makes it hard to select someone who can adequately guide and support you. Another junior faculty member may feel competitive with you and threatened by you, even though he or she has one or two more years of experience. A more senior person may have problems of his or her own, and may consciously or unconsciously try to manipulate you.

REALITY SHOCK

Reality shock is the term used to describe that experience when your expectations are challenged by reality. It is a state of confusion and disorientation in which you are unsure of what behaviors are appropriate. Reality shock occurs when you have accommodated as many discrepancies as you can tolerate between what you expected and what is actually happening. Reality shock can be compounded, too, by other factors. For example, you may have recently moved to a new place where you have few if any friends. Isolation from your previous reference groups while you become a part of a new group of people can be very distressing.

I had been at one institution for over 15 years before entering my present position. It was in a city where I had lived since I was a senior in high school. Although none of my family lived there, I had many deep and long friendships with people both at work and away from work. When I moved, I went hundreds of miles away to a place where I knew no one, except for those I met during my interview! To compound this stress, two of my three cats died within a week after I moved.

Thankfully, I did have a very good idea of what my job would be like, and most of my expectations were met. The faculty and dean were friendly, welcoming, and supportive. However, in my previous position, most of my one-on-one contacts had been with people I knew. In the new position, I was not only dealing with an entire new set of colleagues, but I needed to interview several prospective students each week. I soon felt overloaded with so many new situations and new people. This activity took a lot of energy, and I hadn't expected how much that would drain me.

At the beginning of the school year, there were new activities—receptions, luncheons, meetings, and parties—for the faculty. These felt less like social events than like more demands on my energy. Finally, on a day when the faculty was supposed to attend a reception at the university president's home, I reached my limit. One of the insiders who had already become my friend insisted that I go home and not to the reception. The dean backed her up, and I felt relieved. Of course, I eventually made new circles of friends and became a part of other groups, but those first months were difficult.

The most adaptive thing to do is to get help to sort through what you need and what you don't need. A helpful insider can assist you in this activity, as my new friend did in the situation I just described. People sometimes forget how difficult it can be to be the "new kid on the block," or they may never have experienced it because they have gone from one situation to another that is familiar. Someone with similar experience may be better able to help you to talk about how you're feeling.

ADAPTATION

During the phase of adaptation, the newcomer gradually evolves into an insider. The stages of this process have been described in a variety of works (Freedman, 1979; Locasto & Kochanek, 1988; Ralph, 1978). I have given these stages the following names and describe them based on my experiences and readings:

1. Entry: The novice views the role and nature of the work in a simplistic manner. The role is enacted in a conventional way based on the novice's perceptions of the group's expectations.

2. Differentiation: The novice begins to appreciate the complexities of the role and differentiates the self from the expectations of the group.

3. Diversification: The developing faculty member develops more of a sense of the flexibility and possibilities for change within the setting. Anxiety emerges as the faculty member becomes aware of the true demands of the role. Outrage may occur as the faculty member perceives discrepancies between values and reality.

4. Emergence: The faculty member develops a sense of freedom with the clarification of a personal way of functioning and the tasks involved in the role.

5. Enactment: The faculty member has a clearly developed view of the role. Contradiction and ambivalence are acknowledged and tolerated. The faculty member has a broad view of the role, not only as a member of one group of faculty, but as an educator.

6. Involution: This stage may not be experienced by all faculty members. Disillusionment or other factors may cause the faculty member to turn inward and fail to enact the previously developed role effectively.

As with all developmental processes, each individual moves at her or his own pace. You will encounter people who are fixated in one stage or another, but most continue to evolve and soon reach the stage of enactment. This doesn't mean that they never have any problems of role conflict or role confusion. It merely means that they have matured enough as faculty members to be more tolerant of change, and to participate more effectively in situations demanding their flexibility. Under stressful or unusual circumstances, even a relatively healthy and well developed faculty member may have problems functioning. With support, they can resume their previous role activities.

CONCLUSION

Orienting to a new position is challenging, whether you are new to academia or a seasoned professional. Knowing what to anticipate within the experience will allow you to meet this challenge gracefully. It is a normal human response to try to make sense out of new situations. If you realize that this sensemaking can be affected by your past experiences, you can analyze the new situation and respond more appropriately when you're surprised.

REFERENCES

Freedman, M. (1979). *Academic culture and faculty development.* Berkeley, CA: Montaigne Press.

Locasto, L. W., & Kochanek, D. (1988) Reality shock in the nurse educator. *Journal of Nursing Education, 28,* 79–81.

Louis, M. R. (1980). Surprise and sense making: What newcomers experience in entering unfamiliar educational settings. *Administrative Science Quarterly, 25,* 230–231.

Ralph, N. B. (1978) Faculty development: A stage conception. *Improving College and University Teaching, 26,* 61–63, 66.

THREE

Understanding Politics, Power, and Influence

• •

Politics, power, and influence are part of any human group, and a university and a school of nursing are not exceptions. To function within such a group, you need to understand these concepts and related principles. If you think these are dirty words or things that don't concern you, sooner or later, you're going to get into trouble. As in other things, the best defense is often a good offense. Regardless of your aspirations in academia, you must be aware of the significance of politics and power in human groups.

Learning about the politics, power, and influence in your organization is an important part of becoming a member of that organization. It is crucial to understanding why certain things either do or don't happen. Furthermore, you need to understand these concepts within your specific situation so that you can effectively participate in or initiate change.

PURPOSES

This chapter will help you to:

* define and describe politics, power, and influence;

- use your understanding of politics to help you to be an effective faculty member; and
- identify power and influence strategies which you can use.

POLITICS

Politics is the art or science of influencing the development of policy. Such is Webster's simple definition of the term. Frequently, people imbue the word with an air of deviousness or other unwholesome notions. However, "politics" is merely a word we use to describe the actions and interactions between people determining policies. Universities and schools of nursing are complex organizations in which politics are bound to emerge.

As long as there are differences between people, there will always be politics. The influences that determine policy are bound to exist when people have differing values, priorities, skills, needs, and interests. If you are a part of an institution that values research, in which rewards are more likely to be forthcoming to those who produce research, your beliefs and values will have a greater effect if you fit into that value system. That's politics. In such a system, if you do not have an earned doctorate and have not produced research, your opinions and contributions will often be treated as having less value. Even though you may be a fine teacher who consistently earns good evaluations from students, if you are not a researcher, your voice will be heard less.

In some institutions, the politics dictate that it's not what you know, it's who you know. If you are in favor with the right people, you will have input into policy development. If you are not, your opinions may be undervalued or ignored.

POWER

Power is the capacity to modify the behavior and actions of others without having one's own conduct modified. Power and those who have it are usually apparent to those of us who are veterans of academia. However, it may take a while for a novice to the realm to determine where the different types of power reside.

TYPES OF POWER

If you are interested in the concept of power, I recommend that you read some of the many useful resources on it. A few of these are listed at the end of the chapter. This discussion will touch on only a portion of the framework which may be the most useful to you as you consider the relevancy of power in your situation.

There are four types of power relevant to the organization of schools of nursing. These are: traditional, legitimate, expert, and referent power.

Traditional power is related to beliefs based in the past, in precedents handed down from one generation to the next. Much of this type of power is based on the sanctity of order. This is what gives the existing structure so much influence in most situations. The people who have been around the longest, and people in traditionally powerful positions, have power simply because they have persisted for a long time.

Legitimate power is that which is given to someone by the organization and is accepted and recognized by its members. Examples of this type are those roles which usually carry titles indicating power, such as dean, director, associate dean, coordinator, team leader, and so on.

Expert power is based on one's individual skills, knowledge, and abilities. This power is held by people who have earned certain degrees, had particular experiences, or have accomplished certain outcomes, such as completing research. Although expert power is most significant when it is relevant to the situation, some people have more power in other situations unrelated to their specific expertise. For example, a physician may have more power than a nurse in a faculty meeting regardless of the matter under consideration.

Referent power develops when a person serves as a role model for others. For example, a more experienced faculty member may provide direct and indirect support to new faculty members which helps those people to become more effective in the school. This role gives the experienced faculty member power in dealing with the faculty in two ways. First, the newer faculty members may defer to their experienced colleague. Second, the newer faculty members may subscribe to the values and goals of their role model and provide support for that person's efforts.

As a new, inexperienced faculty member, you will usually have little power. You need to be realistic about this and not expect to have influence before you have paid your dues. That means that you must get the experience and show that you have something to offer. Even if you have a newly earned Ph.D., you still need to prove yourself.

To earn power, you need to assess the organization. You need to gather information by asking the following questions:

1. Using the typology given above, *who already has power?* You cannot earn power if you try to encroach on someone else's area of influence. This would be professional suicide for someone new to an organization. You need to respect the current power structure and understand how it is organized.

2. *How did those people get into those positions of power?* Understanding this will help you to be aware of the ways power can be earned and connections made within the organization.

3. *How are decisions made?* The way in which decisions are made reflects how the power structure really works. You may find that even though a person has a seemingly powerful title, she or he actually has little authority to make decisions. Their superiors may actually set policies while that person is merely expected to carry them out.

4. *Is there a power void in some area?* One way to earn power is to fill a void. For example, if there is no one on the faculty with educational expertise in curriculum development, you may gain power if you have taken a significant number of courses in that field. If you are the only faculty member with a comprehensive understanding of statistics, this may give you some power in situations pertaining to research and development.

5. *What are the values and goals operating within the organization?* To earn power, your activities need to take place within the established value structure. The more your skills and activities are related to institutional goals, the easier it will be to extend your power base. For example, if writing and completing research is highly valued, you will become more powerful if you achieve in these areas.

EARNING POWER

Once you have made an assessment of your organization's structure, you can decide how to direct your professional activities towards becoming a part of that structure. You should consider the following principles in your activities:

1. Be Prepared

There are few things that make as good an impression as being ready to do what needs to be done. This very simple statement, "be prepared," encompasses almost every aspect of your role as a faculty member. It includes the obvious requirement that you be prepared to do your teaching responsibilities. If you are unprepared, your evaluations will reflect this, and you will suffer for it.

You must also be prepared for your other responsibilities, such as attending meetings. If you receive material in advance of a meeting, be sure you read and understand it in advance. Never meet with a colleague or a superior without some preparation. If it's appropriate, have some notes already prepared about the matter to be discussed. Jot down some questions to ask. Sketch some objectives, if that's relevant. These behaviors will not only help you focus on the concerns at hand; they will reflect well upon you as well.

I was once part of a committee interviewing faculty members for a course coordinator position. Two candidates were very similar in terms of education and experience. The one factor that helped us to differentiate between them was that one came prepared and the other didn't. The one who was prepared had already done a lot of homework about what would be involved in the new role. She had some ideas about how she would approach her responsibilities and some goals she hoped to accomplish. In contrast, the other person presented an attitude of "I know I can do it, just give me a chance." The first candidate was obviously the better choice. In addition, she had a history of being well prepared which was known within the school.

2. Build Networks

In addition to your friends at work, you need networks. These may include friends as well as people who have responsibilities connected to yours. You need to nurture relationships with others in your work setting including other teachers, contacts above and below you in terms of responsibility, and contacts outside your school. Information is a valuable commodity in any situation, and one way to increase your access to information is to be in networks where information is shared. In this way you can become aware of possible changes while they are still under consideration. This may help you in following the first principle described above: to be prepared.

The more people who know you, the better it may be for you if you are trying to achieve something. For example, if you want to propose a change which has potentially far-reaching effects on others around you, your views will be more likely to get a hearing if these people know who you are. If you seem to be coming out of nowhere, people may not even listen to what you are proposing.

You need to get to know people outside your organization. For example, if you know other teaching faculty in similar nursing programs, this will help you to be aware of a broader perspective. It may be helpful, when you're proposing something innovative, if you know either who else is doing it or that no one else is doing it.

You need contacts in the clinical areas and in community agencies. This will keep you apprised of developments in those areas as well as provide resources when you need them. This may also give you opportunities to become involved in influencing their policies.

3. Choose Your Issues Carefully

Don't make an issue out of something you can't possibly change. For example, if you are a young faculty member who will be considered for tenure, you need to follow the set guidelines for this process. Don't try to change the entire tenure system while you're being considered yourself. You will waste energies that you should be devoting to the activities that will count.

Don't choose an issue which will earn you powerful enemies, no matter how righteous you feel your cause is. Do select important things to be involved in. Be willing to compromise and collaborate in reaching desired outcomes. Be realistic about a power struggle. The less powerful you are, the more likely it is that you will have to give up more than those with more power. The person with more power is most likely to win. That is why people want power, and that is why it is legitimate for you to work to earn it.

4. Make a Good Impression

Some of this fourth principle is inherent in the previous three. If you are well prepared, have an effective network of contacts, and choose your battles wisely, this will make you look good. You also need to be aware of the values within the organization which are related to the less formal structure. For example, the less power you have, the more you have to look like you're expected to look. If the standard practice is to wear suits or dresses to work rather than more casual clothing, you must dress that way. If you're expected to have an uncluttered office, you must put the time into keeping your work space looking as expected. If being on time is important, and it usually is, you must plan to meet time requirements and make appropriate arrangements if you can't.

Don't ask stupid questions. The best way to avoid this is to be prepared and keep up with what is under discussion. For example, I think it is a minimal requirement for a faculty member in a school of nursing to be familiar with the licensing exam the graduates will take. I have found myself aghast at relatively experienced faculty members who do not know what kind of content is and is not on the NCLEX-RN. Faculty members who do not have this kind of information reduce their own credibility in my eyes. It makes me wonder if they are sloppy about keeping up with their other responsibilities.

5. Have a Voice and Have Something to Say

All the foregoing might make you think that "Mum's the word." However, being too cautious or too reticent is just as counterproductive as doing the wrong thing. You should respond to discussions and memos where your opinion is relevant. Even a new faculty member has plenty to offer. Check with your role models, or faculty who are only a little less new than you, for guidance in participating.

INFLUENCE

Influence is the ability to produce an effect without apparent exertion of force or exercise of authority. It takes place in indirect and intangible ways which are not part of the published organizational chart.

Influence is the subtlest of the three major concepts discussed in this chapter. A person must have power in order to have influence, yet one can have a great deal of influence in a situation where one has little direct power. For example, where a group of faculty has adopted a nursing theorist's model, that theorist might have considerable influence, even though she has no role in the organization itself. The power of the nursing theorist in this case is expert power.

On the other hand, some people may have a great deal of legitimate power due to their positions, but they have limited influence due to other factors. For example, I knew of an assistant dean who was the director of an undergraduate program. He had the power due his role. However, he had little influence, because his faculty did not see him as having the knowledge or expertise to lead them effectively. Faculty members sometimes completely ignored him when making significant decisions. He was eventually relieved of his position.

The main effect of influence is that those with influence are heeded when they express their opinions. Their information is considered to be relevant and is used in making decisions. Those who maintain their positions of influence do so with several strategies:

1. Information Control

People who are influential control the information that goes to the decision makers. They may hold back or emphasize parts of the information in a way that affects the outcome.

2. Expertise

To be influential, a person must possess some expertise of value to those who are being influenced. For example, if you are the faculty advisor to the nursing students' organization, you can expect to have more influence in deliberations pertaining to such extra-curricular activities than someone who did not hold such a position.

3. Effectiveness

You must be effective in what you do in order to have influence. No matter what your credentials are, if you can't deliver what is expected, you will lose your influence. For example, if you never do any research beyond your doctoral dissertation, your ability to affect matters regarding research will decrease each year.

4. Identification

If decision makers identify with you, you will have greater influence with them. For example, when sharing information, you should emphasize the similarities you have to those who are making decisions. If you are perceived as sharing their values and point of view, this will increase the importance of your contributions.

POWER AND INFLUENCE SKILLS

All of the principles described above indicate things you can do to establish a power base for yourself as a faculty member. In addition, there are some other strategies you can use to increase your power and influence.

NETWORKING

I cannot emphasize this strategy too much. You must become part of existing networks and build new ones. Keep your networks healthy by making periodic contacts with the people in them. When you have the chance to show your appreciation or share something with others in your networks, be sure to do so. You have to foster these relationships not only by seeking information of use to you, but by sharing information of use to others.

Frequently, faculty members form too small a support group for themselves. They align themselves with a few people within their clinical area and have few contacts with other nursing faculty, let alone faculty outside the school. You will have more influence if you get to know a variety of your colleagues.

MEDIATING

One way to earn power and establish influence is by facilitating agreement within groups. You may be able to do this when an issue is one on which you are neutral. Even when you hold a strong opinion, you may be able to behave objectively enough to facilitate a resolution of a problem with as few difficulties as possible. By being respectful and helpful in assisting in this way, you earn respect.

Mediating is a skill in which you help two or more diverse groups arrive at a mutually agreeable solution. The most ideal result is a *win-win* situation. In a win-win solution, all parties involved feel they have gotten a good result, regardless of its similarity or dissimilarity to their original goals.

You can often foster this attitude by helping the people on each side of an issue learn to understand and appreciate the ideas of the others. One method is to ask each party to describe and explain the *other side* of the issue. By doing so, they can better appreciate each other's point of view.

Strong emotions can be generated in a disagreement among colleagues. In order for each person to hold to their own belief systems, much antagonism may have developed. You can help by doing something to discharge these unhealthy negative feelings. Situation 3.1 describes a way of doing this.

BEING EFFECTIVE

When you are responsible for something, you need to discharge this responsibility in the most effective way possible. Failure to do this will detract from your influence. The newer you are and the fewer your opportunities to show what you can do, the more pressure there will be on you to do well.

Make sure you know what is expected of you. Know the relevant parameters, such as time limits and paperwork expectations. Don't procrastinate. Ask for help from an experienced colleague if you need it.

INFORMING

Keep your closest associates and your immediate supervisors informed of the information within your control. For example, if

Situation 3.1.

Sharing Appreciations[1]

Our faculty members were deeply divided over an issue related to the curriculum. Discussions and arguments had been going on for a long time and negative feelings on both sides of the issue were running high. Martha Primeaux, the assistant dean, my colleague, Clare Delaney, and I were concerned that this issue was becoming so divisive it would have a negative effect on the group lasting far beyond the specific issue. We were close to the point where the issue needed to be resolved, and we were worried about the final phase of discussion and voting.

Clare and I suggested to Martha that we start the next faculty meeting off with an exercise we used frequently in group exercises with students. The exercise is called "Sharing Appreciations." In this exercise, each participant has a blank piece of paper pinned to her or his back. Everyone is given a felt tipped marker. At this point, everyone in the group circulates around the room and writes one thing on every other person's sheet of paper which describes something they appreciate about that person. After all have done this, each person gets to read what the others wrote about them.

When we told the group we were going to do this, they responded with less than a cooperative attitude. Martha gently chided them and said she wasn't going to start the meeting until we did this. At first, people moved about in an awkward way, and sought out their compatriots on the bothersome issue first. Finally, people had to start going to the people "on the other side." By the time the activity ended, the mood in the room was noticeably different.

Clare and I processed the experience with the others, asking how they felt. Even though they knew we were guiding them to try to get in touch with their good feelings about each other, our faculty members reported having a positive experience. They admitted that it had been a while since they had consciously had good feelings about everyone else.

When we finally began discussing the volatile issue, everyone was much more reasonable and receptive than they had been previously. The group started working in a much healthier fashion, and finally resolved the issue in a way acceptable to almost everyone.

Not only did we accomplish the short-term objective of helping the group over this rough spot, we also earned a lot of respect from our colleagues for what we were able to do. Both of us were frequently asked to make similar interventions or advise on such interventions in the future.

---

[1]"Sharing Appreciations" is an exercise developed by Victoria Schoolcraft and Clare Delaney in 1979 for use in a course at the University of Oklahoma College of Nursing.

you know of an incident that might lead to someone's contacting the dean, let the dean know what you know about it in a timely fashion. One of the most disconcerting things that can happen to a person is to be caught off guard by an irate student or parent. Your influence will be extended if you can help to protect people from being put in embarrassing situations for which they're unprepared.

LEADING

When you have the opportunity to be a leader, do your best. This may take place on a small scale, such as a subcommittee of a standing committee, or on a larger scale, such as a task force for a self-study report. To be effective at leading, you must be well organized, understand your goals, and be able to stimulate your followers to work with you to reach your goals.

INITIATING

Establishing a sense of yourself as an effective initiator of change will give you more influence. To establish this reputation, you need to start in an arena of reasonable scope. For example, choose an issue that affects only you and a few other people. Don't select something about which there is a lot of emotional attachment or that is threatening to others. Choose an issue you know a lot about and can describe effectively to others.

If you time your attempt at change initiation well, and introduce it carefully enough, not only will you make a worthwhile contribution, but you will begin to develop a favorable reputation for yourself. Situation 3.2 describes an incident in which the faculty member gave insufficient consideration to the system she was trying to change. Situation 3.3 describes a more effective attempt.

CONCLUSION

Schools and universities are political in nature. The more you understand and accept this, the better able you will be to function effectively in these arenas. Skills that lead to power and influence can be cultivated, but they take time and effort to put into practice.

Situation 3.2

An Ineffective Attempt at Change

Louise Barber (not her real name) was a recent doctoral graduate with expertise in curriculum development. Although she had no more preparation in testing and evaluation than most doctoral students, she felt she was an expert compared to the rest of her faculty colleagues. One of her doctoral faculty had been an advocate of using "z" scores for determining student grades on tests. Dr. Barber decided to try to convince her new colleagues to adopt this approach.

She initially had influence due to her doctoral preparation, and she seemed to understand what she wanted to do when she approached the assistant dean for the undergraduate program. She arranged to present her proposal to the faculty. However, her presentation was garbled and confusing. She could not adequately explain why her method would minimize bias in assigning grades, or do anything else that seemed worthwhile enough to make a change.

Finally, Dr. Barber resorted to demanding that the faculty accept her proposal just because she knew it was better. The more strident and pompous she became, the less the other faculty members were willing to listen to her. Even though some course coordinators attempted to try the method she recommended, they were frustrated because she was not able to adequately help them to implement it and explain its use to students. They finally returned to the conventional method of using percentages.

Dr. Barber lost the tentative respect she had initially held due to her education. Later, when she tried to use her true expertise, the other faculty members were not receptive. Eventually, she became so frustrated by her lack of influence that she left that school and found a position elsewhere.

Situation 3.3

An Effective Attempt at Initiating Change

Early in my teaching career, I was on the faculty of a college with an integrated curriculum. There were 16 different faculty members with students in clinical areas within one course. Several of us were concerned about the consistency of clinical grading from one person to another.

My colleague, Clare Delaney, and I decided to design a contract for use in clinical grading. We did not introduce the idea as something we thought all faculty members should do, but as a pilot project. We described what we had in mind at a meeting of all the clinical faculty and essentially asked their blessings to try the project.

We needed to keep our colleagues informed so that they would be able to respond if their clinical students questioned the difference between the two systems of grading. We made it clear that we wanted our system considered for use in all clinical practicums, but that we wanted to try the pilot to see if it would be workable.

Clare and I completed our plans, implemented the project, evaluated it, wrote a report, and presented our report to our colleagues. We stated that we wanted to continue using this method and suggested they consider joining us. We allowed lots of time for questions, discussion, and deliberation outside of meetings.

Clare and I were well prepared in all our efforts at making change. We had lots of good, well-organized references to share. We kept good notes on what we did and spent a lot of time thinking of possible concerns or objections before talking with other faculty members. If people were threatened or worried about our method, we responded in a supportive manner, understanding that this was a big change for some people. We emphasized the advantages of this method for both faculty and students. We always treated our colleagues respectfully and sincerely asked for their input.

After many discussions and much consideration, the faculty voted to try this method for one semester. Clare and I did most of the work in designing and preparing all the materials for the process. We also oriented the new students to the system. Since this was their first clinical course, they had no previous experience of being graded in any other way. Although there were problems, things went well enough that this method of clinical grading was adopted and was used for many years.

The effective way in which Clare and I handled this project gave each of us a lot of influence in later situations where we were involved with bringing about change. Although you can do such things alone, my experience with Clare showed me that it can be very helpful to have a partner to work with on projects such as this.

REFERENCES

Bullough, V. L., & Bullough, B. (1984). *History, trends, and politics of nursing*. Norwalk, CT: Appleton-Century-Crofts.

Schorr, T. M., & Zimmerman, A. (1988). *Making choices, taking chances*. St. Louis: Mosby.

Wieczorek, R. R. (1985). *Power, politics, and policy in nursing*. New York: Springer Publishing Co.

Communicating Effectively

•••••••••••••••••••••••••••••••

Being a faculty member means working and communicating with others: students, colleagues, and administrators. Frequently, these communications are oral. Since we talk to people daily and have been talking to people all our lives, we often forget or ignore how complex this process can be. Your abilities as a faculty member will be enhanced by being an effective oral communicator. Chapter 11 will address effective communication in writing.

Some of the situations in which you will need to present information orally include faculty, committee, and professional meetings; ceremonial events; and research presentations. Frequently, the way you say what you have to say is just as important as what you say. The context in which you speak has as much of a bearing on your presentation of information as does the content.

PURPOSES

This chapter will help you to:

- diagnose the strengths and weakness of your oral communication;

- identify the appropriate style of communication in terms of the type or presentation, the group involved, and the context; and
- plan, carry out, and evaluate your oral presentations.

PUBLIC SPEAKING

Although the "public" you are addressing may be a small group of your colleagues, an ability to speak as effectively as if it were a large group of strangers will help you to convey your message. If you have ever taken a speech course, you might review what you learned there. If you haven't taken such a course, you might give it a try. Many colleges and universities offer not only traditional courses in speech, but also evening classes specifically tailored to adult students. This arena will give you the opportunity to learn and to try out well-validated approaches in a safe setting.

This chapter cannot substitute for a speech course, but some of the methods taught in such courses will be discussed here. Of course, simply reading this information is not enough. You will need to plan opportunities to practice the skills outlined here.

ORGANIZATION

Some speaking activities require a certain style of organization. For example, a research presentation usually follows a standard format. If a certain manner of organization is expected and/or required in a particular situation, follow it fairly closely. Otherwise, you may lose some of your audience who are perplexed by being unable to follow you.

On the other hand, you might want to introduce a creative, innovative approach to increase attention and understanding on the part of your audience. Many people give very boring speeches, apparently because that is the model they have usually seen. Use your negative experiences in listening to speeches as a model of what *not* to do. You can enliven a presentation by not doing the predictable thing. For example, start with a colorful illustration of your principal point and use this theme throughout as you proceed according to a logical structure.

This logical way to proceed is probably already familiar to you. Start with a brief introduction to explain what you'll be addressing. You might share the goals or objectives of your presentation. As you proceed with the body of your talk, you can emphasize the important points you're making by designating them consistently with terms such as: points, principles, rules, issues, concerns, problems, hopes, warnings, guidelines, or lessons. You can think of many other words which would better suit some of the things you speak about.

When you're concluding, it is often helpful to sum up main points or give another illustration to pull together the points you have made. However, some speeches have a greater impact if you simply stop and sit down.

STYLE

Style is a highly individual component of any presentation, for your style is influenced by your *personality*. It is also affected by your comfort level in speaking to any given group, as well as by the nature of your presentation. You probably can't change your personality, but you can work on becoming more at ease in doing things which depart from the way in which you see yourself.

Surprisingly, introverts are not necessarily uncomfortable in front of groups. For example, I am somewhat of an introvert when I am dealing with one or two strangers in an informal setting. However, when I get in front of a group of almost any size and have a designated area to cover within my expertise, I am able to forget myself and focus on doing the best I can at getting my message across. Some other introverts have equal difficulty in talking to any number of people, no matter how interested or competent these speakers are in regard to their topics. Conversely, I know people who are very extroverted and are quite good at making others comfortable in unstructured situations. However, some of them are very uncomfortable in front of large groups, even when talking about some of their greatest interests.

My point is that no matter what your personality type, you can be an effective speaker to groups. Don't count yourself out because you're shy or because you've had difficulties in the past. The only way to change is to decide that change is worthwhile and do the appropriate things to institute that innovation.

Your *comfort level* in speaking may vary with the group. You might feel the most comfortable in talking to people who are most similar to your students. Some speakers feel uncomfortable talking to people of a different generation than themselves. You are likely to be more uncomfortable the first time you talk to a certain kind of group. For example, if you are presenting research findings at a national meeting for the first time, you are likely to be nervous, no matter how worthy your material is or how well prepared you are. This is normal. Most people listening to you will want to be supportive; they are interested in knowing what you have to say, or they wouldn't be there. Later in this chapter, I'll address problems that occasionally arise and give some suggestions as to how you might deal with them.

The *nature* of your presentation has an impact on your style. For example, the way you address a formal class is different than the way you give a speech. However, one refuge of teachers who are insecure about public speaking is to treat every oral presentation as if it were a class. Depending on your teaching style, this may or may not be a good idea. A pedantic teaching style may turn off listeners who are, in most respects, your colleagues. However, some teachers use an andragogical approach to their classes which carries over well into other situations. "Andragogy" is a term coined by Malcolm Knowles (1980) to describe the process of teaching adults. This concept has wide applications which are pertinent to communications. Andragogy will be discussed further later in this chapter.

Speech Skills

Before you open your mouth, your *appearance* will speak for you. Take care to look right for the event. Dress like a professional person. If you're going to be on a stage in a large room or auditorium, wear something that will show up well, such as clothing with bright colors. It's especially helpful in these situations to wear something that is bright and draws attention to your face, such as a colorful scarf or a bright necktie. If you know what the background of your speaking platform will be like, be sure to wear clothes that will contrast with it so you don't seem to be blending in. Check your hair and make-up before starting.

Speak at a *pace* that is slow enough for people to understand you, but not so slow that your audience is restless for you to finish. One of the biggest distractions in public speaking is an awareness of how fast or how slow the speaker is talking. Try tape recording your speech and listen to the pace. You may be surprised at what you hear.

Speak in a well modulated *tone*. Be careful about lapsing into a monotone. Sometimes you may want to emphasize a point by speaking more loudly than usual or by speaking very softly. As suggested above, you can assess your ability to vary your tone by reviewing tape recordings.

If needed, use a *microphone* to amplify your speech. There is nothing more frustrating for an audience than straining to hear a speaker. If what you have to say is important, people will forget that your voice is being mechanically amplified. However, if they can't hear you well, that is all they will remember.

Stay on your feet and *move* around as much as you can without feeling awkward. Even stepping to one side or the other of the podium may help to stimulate your listeners.

Use *gestures* to emphasize points, but avoid using distracting mannerisms. To help you evaluate your skills in this area, have yourself videotaped and replay it while turning off the sound.

Make *eye contact* with various people in your audience. *Smile* appropriately, being careful not to smile if it might imply a lack of concern for someone or something you're discussing.

Use *anecdotes* carefully. You can alter anecdotes in order to make them concise enough to make your point. Make sure that people understand what point you're trying to make with your story. I have a vivid memory of an inappropriate anecdote told at the baptism of my goddaughter. The day should have been up-beat, but the minister told an anecdote about symbols which in-volved someone dying in a meaningless way. Make sure your anecdote is not only appropriate in terms of content, but also in terms of feeling.

If you use *jokes*, make sure they don't seem to deprecate any-one. Don't use off-color or suggestive material. Sometimes a hu-morous story is easier to tell than a joke per se.

If you *quote* lengthy passages, make sure it's worth the time; it may work better to paraphrase. Be sure to give credit appropri-ately.

Convey *enthusiasm*. Let people know that you care about your topics by using a lively *vocabulary* and an *expressive face*. Know how

much *time* you're supposed to take and stay within the boundaries.

Use your *anxiety* to motivate you to do better in the future. One
of my students once gave a presentation and was obviously very
anxious. She suddenly stopped, took a deep breath, and admitted she was nervous. Then she asked if we would give her a
smile to remind her we were her friends. The group responded
with big, genuine smiles, and she visibly calmed down.

DEALING WITH PROBLEMS

There are three different sources of problems you encounter in an
oral presentation: yourself, other people, and things.

Problems originating with you would include those relating to
organization, style, and time. People have different methods of
organization. The way I organize a speech may seem a lot different
than yours, but both methods may work. You may make problems for yourself by being inadequately prepared or poorly organized. It's hard to make up for poor organization while you're in
the midst of the presentation. You can learn from this experience
for the future, but you may not be able to fix the problem on the
spot.

Your *style* may present problems if it turns out to be unsuitable
for the context. If you like to walk up and down the aisles while
you talk, this may distract some people or it may be undesirable
because your voice cannot be heard by all. If you intend to encourage audience participation, but the group is unreceptive to
this, you could end up with a big hole in your plans. Monitor the
situation carefully and be able to change your style if your favored
method is impractical.

Timing may also become an issue if you don't manage it well
while you're speaking, or if you don't adequately set limits on the
participation of others involved. Most experienced speakers are
able to figure out how to cut down their presentations even while
they're talking.

It's sometimes necessary to expand on what you're saying. You
can sometimes use extra time to elaborate on shorter examples,
or to add content you originally thought you wouldn't have time
for. Conversely, you may create problems by getting bogged
down and spending too much time on some aspect of your pre-

sentation to the detriment of other parts. Adhering to time constraints will improve the impression you make.

Other people may create difficulties in a variety of ways. Questions, for example, can be a problem if handled incorrectly. Although they signify interest in your topic, the participants may interrupt to such an extent that it disrupts the flow of your presentation. If this becomes a problem, ask them to hold their questions until the end of the talk. Be sure you structure your presentation so that ample time remains for these questions.

Sometimes, you may just have hit the group on a bad day. For reasons beyond your control, they may be distracted or uninterested in what you have to say. This may be manifested by restlessness and noise. It is usually appropriate to graciously ask for quiet. You may be able to recapture the group's interest by asking for more involvement on their part. Getting them to think of an application of what you're saying, or asking for input, may perk their interest. Most groups will at least be polite, even if they're not completely impressed with you.

Some people may unintentionally put you on the spot by asking a question you can't answer. This may be embarrassing, but it's usually better to admit you can't answer the question than to try to fake it. In some situations you may want to stall while you try to come up with a rejoinder. You may ask the questioner for a response, or ask for comments from the rest of the group. This will give you some time to gather your own thoughts. Keep in mind that resorting too much to this tactic will tend to make you look less genuine. Before you're ever confronted with this, think of how you would deal with a difficult question.

Occasionally, you may be greeted by overtly negative responses. People make facial expressions or in other nonverbal ways demonstrate that they don't agree with you or don't like what you're saying. Some people may challenge you openly and try deliberately to put you on the spot. This generally occurs when your topic is controversial. Knowing this allows you to prepare in advance for unpleasant responses. Think about how you would respond to such negativity before it happens. Remember, if you lose your cool, you'll lose your opportunity to have any influence.

The things that can create problems for you include everything from the temperature of the room and outside noises beyond your control, to problems with furniture or the sound system, or to power failures. If you can exert some control to change or stop problematic factors such as these, do so as quickly as possible. If you cannot eliminate the disturbance, it is handled best by acknowledging it and engendering a feeling that you are as unhappy as your audience about the situation.

When things create problems, humor can help to dissipate tension in the group as well as to relieve your own discomfort. I was once giving a keynote speech at a hotel when suddenly loud music came on over the sound system. It was impossible to talk over the noise, so I asked the participants to play "name that tune" while another person tried to get the music shut off. This prevented both me and the audience from becoming aggravated enough to detract from the speech I was giving.

Another time, I was lecturing in a hall with a stage that thankfully was only a few steps higher than the main floor. While I was still talking, I walked off the stage and fell on the floor. I wasn't hurt but I was startled. The students didn't know whether to laugh or not. However, I knew that laughter usually diminishes the tension of embarrassing moments. I got up, stepped back on the stage, took a bow and said, "For my next trick...." The students and I laughed, and I was able to proceed.

HARD COPY

For most speeches, you will need to have your remarks in some hard format for reference. Unless you are exceptionally good at memorizing, you will rarely have any reason to try it. You should be familiar enough with your speech that you can comfortably speak without reading all of it. However, having the written copy available will ensure that you keep track of what you want to say.

Some people prefer to have their speeches typed, double- or triple-spaced. Others may have them hand-written on paper or cards. I do some of both, depending on the nature of the presentation. A typed speech will probably be easier for you to follow and keep track of where you are. I have sometimes found that I have overlooked points when I've had them hand-written.

Selby, Tornquist, and Finerty (1989b) suggest several things to make the hard copy of your speech more useable.

- Have your speech typed on heavy paper that will not rustle, and slide your pages to the side rather than turning them over;
- If you do not always wear your glasses, use a typeface that you can easily read without them. The best typeface will vary for each person. Choose what works for you;
- Outdent, rather than indent, your paragraphs so that they will be more apparent to you;
- Use highlighters or other methods to draw your attention to key words so you don't forget to use them;
- Don't split words from one line to another, and don't split a sentence between two pages;
- Number the pages, but don't staple them together;
- Mark on your paper points where you want to use a slide or transparency; and
- If you're using a lot of slides, use a separate piece of paper for each one and tape a copy of the slide text to it.

If you use cards, many of the same guidelines apply. I like 5" x 8" cards because they are easy to manipulate, and I can easily add to or take away cards from other presentations. For example, an anecdote on one card could easily be inserted in any group of cards for a given speech. The most important thing is to have them numbered so that you don't get mixed up.

KNOWING YOUR AUDIENCE

Part of the effectiveness of oral communication depends on presenting it appropriately for the recipients. You may have all the most accurate information on the topic, but fail to help the group because you present this information in too complex a fashion or because you seem to be patronizing the audience. Some examples of such problems include:

- using complex, undefined terminology in a class of high school students interested in nursing;
- giving a lecture about the nursing process as a speech at a pinning ceremony;

- describing the nursing process to nursing educators as if they were inexperienced students; and
- giving an unstructured research presentation in a formal research program.

All of the above situations are ones I have seen in my own experience, and you can probably think of several of your own.

When you plan to speak to a group, *identify the members of the potential audience*. At times, this will be evident, as with a faculty or committee meeting or a class of high school students. At other times, the audience may be unpredictable and varied, such as with attendees at a research conference. In the latter situation, the audience may range from inexperienced nursing students to highly experienced nurse researchers. You should find out who usually attends such groups in order to appropriately plan your presentation.

In some situations, your approach may easily be identified. If you are talking to a group of your school of nursing colleagues, you may have a fairly good idea of their level of knowledge and experience with the topic you will address. However, if the prospective audience is made up of faculty beyond the school of nursing, the group may be much more varied, with great strengths in some aspects of what you're discussing and great weaknesses in others. An example of the latter case is given in Situations 4.1 and 4.2.

When you're preparing to speak to groups about whom you know little, don't make assumptions. Talk beforehand to contacts who are familiar with the prospective audience. An example appears in Situation 4.3. I've included this story to show that even if you do plan, you can leave something out. Sometimes something about the group will affect what happens. Another example of such problems is found in Situation 4.4. In that situation, my planning was perfectly appropriate to what I was asked to do and for the anticipated audience. I chose not to modify the presentation on the spot as I had done in Situation 4.3. The content of this speech did not lend itself to being modified for the many inappropriately assigned people there. I wanted to offer what I had for the nurse managers who were there in good faith, and for whom the workshop was intended in the first place. I decided it

Situation 4.1

Grand Rounds

I once gave a presentation at Grand Rounds for the Department of Psychiatry. My topic was Post-Traumatic Stress Syndrome, with a focus on rape victims. At the time, this was a fairly new diagnostic category. Experienced professionals in the field were well aware of the picture presented by some of the clients involved. However, most of the participants had not looked at rape victims as sufferers of such a syndrome and had little experience in dealing with them. I was not only aware of the way rape victims fit into the classification, but I had a wealth of experience gained as a founder and volunteer at the county rape crisis center. I had worked with over 100 recent and not-so-recent victims of rape.

In making my presentation, I needed to briefly review the components of the classification and its use in making a diagnosis. However, since that is usually the physician's responsibility, I spent little time with trying to teach about diagnosis. Instead I put my efforts into describing the women involved and how the classification could be used to intervene with them. It was rare for these professionals to have a nurse present to them, but I felt very well received because I structured my presentation in such a way as not to encroach on what they considered their expertise. I was still able to effectively share my knowledge and skill.

Situation 4.2

Panel Presentation

Public speaking doesn't always run smoothly, even if you think you know your audience. I was once part of a panel that included mostly lay volunteers from the rape crisis center. We presented at Grand Rounds for the Department of Gynecology and Obstetrics. Some of the residents were openly antagonistic toward us since they did not feel we were professionals. One resident stood up and informed us that "half the time" the women who claimed to be raped were lying. I knew it was important not to turn the presentation into a contest about who knew the truth. I simply shared statistics from a variety studies showing how many rapes went unreported and supporting the claim that almost all accusations of rape appeared to be true. I did not argue with the resident, but said that perhaps his experience had been different than these reports. Then we moved on.

Situation 4.3

Promoting Creativity

Several times in the past I have conducted a continuing education workshop called "Promoting Creativity" aimed at registered nurses. A nurse manager in a rural hospital heard about my workshop and invited me to present it at her hospital. Somehow I got the impression that all the participants would be RNs, but I never checked this out. Although the workshop's didactic content is applicable to any group, all my anecdotes and some of the material for the breakout sessions revolved around things only RNs would do. Thankfully, I used a technique I always use with small groups: I asked all the participants to introduce themselves, tell a little about what they did, and say what they hoped to get out of the workshop. I was surprised and dismayed when I discovered only about a third of the 25 participants were RNs. The others were records clerks, housekeepers, maintenance people, food service workers, and about every other kind of worker you find in a hospital who *isn't* a nurse.

This situation certainly tested my ability to *be* creative as well as to facilitate the development of creativity. I revised some of my anecdotes on the spot so that they should have more general application. For the first break-out session, I gave the participants an activity that wasn't related to nursing. While they were working on this, I revised the situational cues for later sessions to make the cues more generic. The group was very responsive and seemed to have no idea that I was recreating my workshop while they were experiencing it. I got great evaluations, which were all the more prized since the participants had to complete them in semi-darkness due to power failure. The participants augmented the dim ambient illumination with matches and lighters. It was a fitting end to a day that proved there is more to light than electricity.

Situation 4.4

Motivating Your Employees

I once was asked to another rural workshop specially designed for nurse managers and called "Motivating Your Employees." The continuing education director who arranged for my presentation knew the intended audience and communicated that to the hospital administrator. However, few nurse managers were available to attend, so the administrator sent some nurses who were not managers, as well as LPNs, aides, ward clerks, and miscellaneous other folk from a variety of departments. My first task was to try to motivate the many people who resented being sent to workshop. They felt (and rightly so) that there was little reason for them to be there.

Some sat in rigid positions throughout the day, took no notes, appeared to be day-dreaming, and refused to participate in break-out sessions. Clearly, I had no authority over them, and I knew it was unrealistic to think I could motivate them in such a brief session and under such unfavorable conditions. I acknowledged their situation in front of the whole group, and I made it clear that motivating people to do something requires some willingness to participate on the part of the person you're trying to motivate. I also made it clear that motivation takes time, and that the content and techniques I planned to share would also take time to be effective. I then essentially gave people permission not to participate if they chose not to. This helped to make it clear that while my focus would be on those who wanted to participate and learn, I would not humiliate or intentionally make the others uncomfortable.

Almost all of those who didn't want to participate maintained their demeanor throughout the day. I think maybe one or two actually began to look interested, but I wouldn't bet on it.

was not my responsibility to try to make up for the poor decision of the administrator who sent the wrong people to the workshop. I thought that administrator should have attended and learned something about the subject.

APPLICATIONS

Among the many situations in which faculty members are asked to speak are: proposals to faculty; recruitment; public addresses; ceremonies; research and paper presentations; and continuing education.

PROPOSALS

When you present a proposal to your colleagues, although the most important thing is for you to be well-prepared in terms of knowing your content, you need to anticipate the responses of your audience. You probably already know some of their strengths and weaknesses. By the same token, you may have developed some biases about them which you've never examined. Ask colleagues to whom you feel close to help you examine the nature of the group. Try to be fair-minded when evaluating your associates. Those who differ from you in their perceptions and responses to situations are the first ones you need to think about satisfying. They may be your toughest critics, so you need to be prepared to meet their expectations and potential criticisms.

If possible, give your colleagues written material in advance. This will help them to be prepared and they won't feel you're trying to push something on them which is entirely new. If appropriate, use handouts or other visual aids to make your proposal clear.

When the time comes to speak, follow the guidelines given earlier in this chapter. Never assume, just because you think your proposal is logical and worthwhile, that everyone else will hold the same opinion. Be prepared for challenges and be ready to meet them with grace and serenity. Becoming upset or defensive when your ideas are challenged will undercut the power of your message.

RECRUITMENT

Although your school or university may have people especially designated as recruiters, you may be called upon to assist in this activity. This may take place in the context of a specific recruiting event or a career day at a high school.

Young People

A speech to high school-aged or younger students requires a variety of things to pique their interest. A conventional speech will not hold their attention for long. You need to rely on other cues to help you get your message across.

Consider going to such events in either a uniform or lab coat. While not everyone likes these costumes, they are easily recognizable symbols that help people to understand what you are. Another alternative is to dress more casually than you might ordinarily, so that there doesn't seem to be as wide a difference between you and the audience as might be the case if you were wearing a suit.

One of my friends who does recruiting sometimes takes a skeleton or lab mannequin with her. Such visual aids attract attention, you can also explain how nursing students use them. Take a stethoscope and sphygmomanometer and allow the students the opportunity to check their own or others' vital signs. Have plenty of handout materials available, showing your campus and, specifically, things relevant to nursing students.

If you have access to well-made videos or slide presentations, use those to augment your speech. It is especially helpful to use media that are geared to the age of your audience. Young people often respond well to visual aids that appeal to their values or their sentimental sides. Videos that feature working with children are particularly useful. Material with an emotional appeal can be very effective; even those young people who do not choose a nursing career may gain a new sense of respect for those who do.

In the course of demonstrating equipment or using media, you can interject the important points you want to make. Be prepared for outrageous questions and unexpected responses, particularly considering the developmental stage of your audience. For example, one friend of mine, the one with the lab mannequin, once participated in a career day for thousands of high school students from all over Miami. Her mannequin was equipped with male genitalia, and one of the high school students flipped the cover off the lower part of the mannequin just as a local television crew was filming in the booths. My friend didn't get embarrassed by this normal adolescent behavior, but joined the students and the camera crew in laughing heartily. She was probably more able to communicate with her audience after these young people saw her natural and accepting response to a situation which might have been embarrassing for some.

It is difficult to talk to young people if you haven't done so for a while. If you try to use their popular slang, you may sound either patronizing or condescending. Don't try to do so unless you really understand their language and can use it comfortably. You may find it helpful to rehearse your presentation before some young people you know or can "borrow" from friends or colleagues. Ask these teenagers to give you their honest responses about how your presentation affects them. They can tell you if kids their age would think what you're saying is interesting, as well as if your talk is presented effectively for people their age.

Adults

Recruiting adult students is usually easier for most of us, since we feel more similar to them. Adults who are interested in your program will want concrete and specific information about what you have to offer them. When you speak to adults, no less than to young people, it is important to give them something they can take away to look at later, such as informative handouts or colorful brochures.

Adults are most interested in things they think they can use immediately. In recruiting adults, start with what they want to know most. For example, in talking to prospective RN to BSN students, I start with the curriculum and go over what these students already have and what they will need to complete their degree. Emphasize the ways in which your program has been modified to suit their needs. Be prepared to explain why some things may be less flexible than some students might like.

In talking to your colleagues who have less education than you do, it is especially important that you convey sincere respect for what they are considering in returning to school. My belief is that we all make the best decisions we can given our situations. Most people who choose to get a diploma or associate degree education first do so for practical reasons. We need to convey to them that we respect their decision and admire them for their new choice to work on the BSN.

When I am recruiting adult students who are not already RNs, I usually start by finding out about them and their motives for considering a nursing career. I try to slant my presentation toward the aspects relevant to their motives. For example, many adults who consider a nursing career do so because they want a more service-oriented career. I emphasize the ways in which nursing can gratify these needs. Some people, equally service-oriented, view nursing as a more secure occupation than their previous career. I try to respond to these pragmatic motives by discussing such things as the mobility and variety within the discipline.

PUBLIC ADDRESSES

Frequently, nurses are asked to speak to civic organizations or other large groups, and act as keynote speakers at professional meetings. At such events, always be aware that whether you like it or not, for some people in the audience, you are representing your entire profession. Take care in what you wear that you project the image of a professional person. Never wear a uniform to such an event unless it is specifically called for—and I can't think of a reason it would be.

Review the guidelines given earlier in the chapter concerning assessment the audience and their individual interests. Be very clear about what the topic is and what you are expected to address. An example of this is given in Situation 4.5.

CEREMONIES

A *ceremony* is defined as a series of acts prescribed by ritual or protocol. A speaker at such an event must address the celebrants in the appropriate context. Ceremonies familiar to nursing faculty

Situation 4.5

Hurricane Andrew

Recently a nurse who had been involved in the relief efforts after Hurricane Andrew struck South Florida was asked to talk about this from the standpoint of a nurse. She was asked to speak to a group of laypeople as well as to a group of nurses. She presented her experiences in a different way to each group. For the lay audience, she emphasized the perspective of the people who were being helped. She encouraged the audience to identify with the plight of those people and to appreciate what the nurses provided in the situation. She helped them to identify ways in which nurses could be of help to them if they ever suffered a similar disaster.

For the nurse audience, the speaker emphasized the nurse's role and specific nursing activities during the disaster relief. Although she also helped them to appreciate the feelings of the victims, her thrust was on developing audience identification with the nurses. She also shared useful information with them to help them to respond in similar disaster situations.

To both groups, the speaker imparted a sense of the dedication and courage of the nurses who helped in the relief efforts. Both audiences were obviously moved by the presentations. The lay audience seemed inspired to admire the nurses; the nurse audience felt pride in their colleagues and in themselves.

include capping, striping, pinning, convocation, and commencement.

Speeches at ceremonies should ideally be short, sweet, and inspiring. Formulate your speech based on the reason for the ceremony. Most ceremonies are related to ending one endeavor and embarking on another for which the first prepared you. One obvious theme for such an occasion is "change and growth."

Typically, the audience includes participants who may be naive about the professional field. Although it might be pleasant to include some "inside" anecdotes or jokes which might only be meaningful to the principals, try to limit these so that others do not feel excluded. A graphic and explicit story characteristic of nursing, for example, might be modified so as not to offend listeners unfamiliar with the topic.

RESEARCH AND PAPER PRESENTATIONS

Presentations of research or scholarly papers are usually very structured. Make sure you are aware of the parameters within which you are to make your presentation. Time limits may be strict and are often enforced unceremoniously. If you are told you have 15 minutes, you must do your best to be finished in that amount of time, or you will be cut off. This can be embarrassing, but it is necessary so that one presenter does not encroach on the time allotment for others.

Selby, Tornquist, and Finerty (1989a) have done an excellent job of describing research presentations. One of the principal points they make is that it is important to focus on the findings and conclusions. You should refer to your review of literature very briefly, if at all. You need only describe your methodology if it is likely to be unfamiliar to your audience. Give much detail on the methodology only if that is the specific intent of the presentation or if you are describing the development of a particular instrument.

The more complex your findings, the more helpful it will be to use slides or transparencies to illustrate what you are saying. Don't ever simply copy a page out of your text, but take the time, effort, and expense to produce well-designed media. Selby, Tornquist, and Finerty (1989b) have nicely described the production of effective slides. The key principle is to keep your slides and transparencies as uncluttered and as easy to see and read as possible. One of the most fundamental rules is that slides and transparencies should have no more than eight lines of text, and there should be no more than six words in a line.

CONTINUING EDUCATION

Although continuing education presentations are basically like other teaching activities, I am including this topic here in order to emphasize some of the principles relevant to working with adult learners. Adults tend to want to learn things that they see as having immediate application for them. Adults are also more likely than children to want to participate in their learning, and are more able to do so in an effective way.

When working with adults in continuing education, you may sometimes choose to lecture to them when you have factual information to impart and to explain. However, other methods, such as seminars, discussion groups, and interactive strategies, are often more effective in keeping them interested. Even though adults may seem to resist interactive teaching-learning strategies, they will usually prefer them to being lectured.

Adult learners tend to want to set their own goals. They want to learn about things which will be immediately relevant to them. These students have life experience which may be relevant to what you're teaching or talking about, and they will want to share their knowledge.

Some adult students immediately respect and appreciate their professors. They accept that if you have your degrees and a faculty appointment, you must know what you're doing. They demonstrate eagerness to learn from you and respond well to class assignments. However, other adult students are more skeptical and require that you prove to them that you know what you're talking about. They may question your assignments and resist participating in class.

For some adults, assuming the student role may make them feel as if they are in a subordinate position to the teacher. As a teacher, you need to recognize defensive behaviors which indicate that the student or students are trying to protect their egos. For example, they may become argumentative or sullen. Don't be defensive and angry, but see these behaviors as signs that the students are threatened. Respond in a supportive way that shows genuine concern for their feelings. Convey to them directly your respect for their decision to return to school, and your understanding of the challenge of the student role.

When you speak to classes of adult students, you need to convey confidence in your own expertise. However, you should do this in a way that doesn't minimize the accomplishments of your students. When I'm teaching a class with RNs, whether they're undergraduates or graduates, these students usually know a lot more than I do within their clinical specialties, unless they're in mental health. Even then, they are experts within their specific work setting. I always make sure they know that I realize and appreciate their competencies. I try to help them identify the knowledge and experience they already have that is relevant to my class.

When you're working with adults, especially RNs, remember that even though they may not be your peers in the same way as are other nurse educators, they are still your colleagues in the professional sense. I find it gratifying to work with adults who already share some of the interests and values I have because they are professional nurses. I honestly admire people who are willing to return to school to earn a degree which will not only enhance their career opportunities, but will also increase their potential to contribute to nursing. I always try to convey this attitude when I am teaching them.

CONCLUSION

As educators, we have many opportunities to speak to groups of colleagues, students, other health professionals, and members of the public. We can foster our speaking skills to do this effectively. Many small skills as well as the obvious large ones contribute to being an effective speaker, and most of these can be learned. Even if we already have skills in this area, we may be able to improve upon them as we become more experienced and comfortable in our roles as educators.

REFERENCES

Farley, J. K. (1990). Enhancing oral presentations through visual images. *Nurse Educator, 15*(5), 3–4.

Knowles, M. S. (1980). *The modern practice of adult education: From pedagogy to andragogy.* Chicago: Follett.

Selby, M. L., Tornquist, E. M., & Finerty, E. J. (1989a). How to present your research: Part I. *Nursing Outlook, 37,* 172–175.

Selby, M. L., Tornquist, E. M., & Finerty, E. J. (1989b). How to present your research: Part II. *Nursing Outlook, 37,* 236–238.

Wlodkowski, R. J. (1985). *Enhancing adult motivation to learn.* San Francisco: Jossey-Bass.

·············· FIVE ··············

Relating to Students

·····································

In addition to teaching students, you also have a myriad of other contacts with them. This includes academic advisement, working with student organizations, and less formal contacts. Some of these situations require specific talents, while others only demand the usual social skills you use in any relationship.

PURPOSE

The purpose of this chapter is to help you to:

- advise students effectively for academic decisions;
- work effectively with student organizations; and
- deal appropriately with students outside the classroom or other formal interactions.

ACADEMIC ADVISEMENT

Although some schools have counselors whose role is dedicated to academic advisement, many faculty members are usually expected to work with students to accomplish this goal. The purpose of academic advisement is to guide students in making sound decisions about their progress.

The complexity of advisement is determined by the nature of the curriculum in your school. For example, in some programs, students must complete their nonnursing requirements prior to starting their nursing courses. In these situations, the students may require little assistance in selecting courses once they enter the nursing curriculum. Their pattern of course work may be predetermined. In other situations, non-nursing and nursing courses may be taken concurrently. Students need assistance in planning a well-balanced course load.

Before starting to work with advisees, you must be aware of the policies governing students in your institution. You need copies of such things as the following:

- University catalog
- School bulletin
- Student handbook
- Faculty handbook

Within these resources, you need to know how to locate policies and procedures which would relate to advising students. Even if you have been advising for a while, you may forget the specifics. It is impossible to have every policy and procedure memorized, but you need to know how to locate relevant information as needed by students.

If you have not done academic advising before, or if you are new to a school, the school may provide an orientation to this activity. If it is not provided, seek out an appropriate person to help orient you to the institution's pattern and procedures. Look at some advising files and discuss the content and the process.

INITIAL CONTACT

When a student is first assigned to you for advisement, you should initiate an advisory meeting. In some schools, this will be initiated for you. For example, students may receive a letter when they are admitted, telling them who their advisors are and how to contact them. In other situations, you may need to make the first contact with your advisees. Table 5.1 shows a letter which might be appropriate for this purpose.

Preparing for the Meeting

Before meeting with a new advisee, review the student's file to make sure it includes whatever is expected given your academic

Table 5.1

Initial Advisory Letter

Dear Ms. Day:

Welcome to the Walker University School of Nursing. You have been assigned to me for academic advisement. According to your file, you have already completed some of your prerequisites at a community college. It appears that you still need the following courses before beginning the nursing courses:

> Human Physiology
> Human Growth and Development
> English Composition II
> Speech
> College Algebra
> Introduction to Probability and Statistics

I am available for advisement and signing registration cards on Mondays and Wednesdays from 2:00–4:00 PM. My office is in the School of Nursing building, room 231. Please call for an appointment at 555–1111. Since school will be starting in just a few weeks, I encourage you to come to see me soon. At that time, we can plan how to complete the above credits and review your program of study.

I will be looking forward to meeting you. I hope you are going to enjoy being a student at Walker.

Best wishes,

Mary Lowe, R.N., Ph.D.
Associate Professor

---

setting. Usually, an advisory file will contain copies of transcripts from the high school and/or colleges attended, an evaluation of credits accepted in transfer, and a program plan of some kind. There will also be a form on which to keep a record of contacts with the student, as well as other notes pertaining to the student's progress. Your school's records may have other components. If the student was required to write an essay or gather references for admission, for example, these will be in the file. A copy of the student's health record is also likely to be included.

Sometimes, the student's program plan is preset. In other words, every student is expected to take the same courses at the same times. However, students frequently start school in one place and transfer to another school for the nursing component. Therefore, they may come to you with a lot of the prerequisites completed, or they may have an unusual combination of credits as compared to your students who started at your university. These students need guidance in properly selecting and enrolling in courses.

Some programs concentrate the nursing courses in the junior and senior year. Before starting those courses, students are expected to have completed all or most of the non-nursing requirements. In other schools, students may start their nursing in the sophomore year and fulfill some of their non-nursing requirements along with the nursing courses. These require more time to advise, so that they will meet all the requirements within the usual time frame of the program.

Many schools offer a variety of options in addition to the basic or generic option, such as transitional programs for RNs seeking their BSNs or accelerated options for second-career students. These students may have different ways of meeting requirements because of their past education. However, a plan of their programs will guide you in guiding them.

First Meeting

At the first meeting, start by introducing yourself and getting to know a little bit about your advisee. Find out if the student already has some concerns or questions that she or he is eager to get answered. Describe what your role is as the advisor, including the responsibilities mandated for you by school or university policy. For example, the university may require an advisor's signature for the student to register for any courses. Even though the student may be well aware of the program plan, the advisor may always be required to give written permission to register. This is a protection for the student, assuring that problems may be avoided or minimized.

Let your advisee know when you are available and how best to reach you. If your school has a student handbook, make sure the student has a copy. In some situations, it may be the advisors' responsibility to see that the students have this resource. You might take some time in your first meeting to go over those parts of the handbook that are most relevant to the student's current situation.

If you are aware of common problems for students in your system, you should draw the student's attention to things that will help to avoid these difficulties. Students often do not realize that practically every contingency is covered by some type of policy. The result is that if a problem arises, they make inappropriate decisions based on erroneous assumptions. For example, a student may have attended a school which had a different way of responding to absences from class. The student may assume that your school's policy would be the same. This could result in that student's receiving a failing grade because of failure to withdraw properly.

Go over what the student has completed and what the student needs to complete. If the institution has a specific pattern for courses, it will help if the student has a copy of this. Discuss what courses will be taken when, and help the student prepare a registration form for the next term. The schedule for a university term usually includes directions about registering as well as a calendar of relevant dates. Make sure the advisee has a copy of this document and realizes the significance of this information. Verify that the advisee understands how to go about registering and when to do it.

Clarify when the student should meet with you again. Make sure your advisee knows when you can be reached if other problems arise during the course of the term.

Follow-up Meetings

Your advisees will need to meet with you periodically as they proceed through their nursing program. At times, these meetings may be perfunctory because the student's course of action has been predetermined. Although it is important that you convey an interest in all your advisees, they may not need a lot of attention once they become accustomed to the program and the university.

Academic Difficulties

You may occasionally need to meet with students due to problems they are having. For example, students in academic difficulty in courses may be required to meet with their advisors. Generally, this need will come to your attention because the faculty member responsible for the course in which the student is enrolled will send you a copy of a formal notice sent to the student. Usually, the student is directed to contact you. Frequently, they are reluctant to do so because they may fear that you will be harsh with them. You may encourage them to meet with you by sending a supportive letter. An example is given in Table 5.2.

When you meet with a student about academic difficulties, there are several things to discuss. Some of the things you might address are:

Table 5.2

Academic Difficulty Letter

Sharon Walsh
Shaw Hall, # 14
Walker University

Dear Sharon:

I received a copy of the midterm grade deficiency report in Physiology that you received from Dr. Bradley. I regret that you are having trouble with this course. Please make an appointment to meet with me to discuss this situation.

It isn't unusual for people to have problems with their courses. One of the reasons you have me for your advisor is to have someone to help you deal with these difficulties. I will work with you to identify methods that may be of help to you so that you can complete this course successfully.

I will be looking forward to meeting with you. I encourage you to see me within the next two weeks.

Sincerely,

Mary Lowe, R.N., Ph.D.
Associate Professor

What Does the Student Think the Problem Is?

Frequently, students have already diagnosed their problems before they meet with you. They often have insight into their difficulties, and this should be reinforced. On the other hand, some students may think they have diagnosed the problem, but in fact they are attributing it to someone else, such as the instructor. Although some instructors may be tougher than others, the student needs to learn how to adapt to increased demands, whether or not these demands seem fair to the student or even to you.

Has the Student Already Started Doing Something to Rectify the Problem?

Students who have already thought about the problem will also often have determined a course of action. This is frequently quite appropriate to the situation. By discussing it with you, as their advisor, they make a firmer commitment to follow through with their plan.

Has the Student Talked With the Instructor?

Sometimes the instructor can help the student to focus on the true nature of the problem. Students are often reluctant to approach an instructor, especially one in whose course they are having difficulty. You can help the student to prepare for such an interaction.

How Are the Student's Note-taking Skills?

Ask the student to show you the notes from the class. Some students have difficulties because they have no idea how to take notes. You may find that their notes are skimpy, poorly organized, difficult to read, or irrelevant. You can give them assistance in learning how to take better notes, or refer them elsewhere for this assistance if it is available within your university. Some students may be helped if they can audiotape lectures and listen to them again while reviewing their notes. Of course, the instructors must give permission for this.

How Are the Student's Reading Skills?

The student may have reading and/or comprehension problems. A quick way to diagnose this is to ask the student to read a passage aloud to you from an unfamiliar book which is within what should be the student's range of comprehension. Then ask the student to explain what she or he just read. If comprehension seems to be a problem, refer the student to the appropriate resource on campus for a more accurate diagnosis and assistance in dealing with reading.

Most adults, even college students of traditional age, are very sensitive about any notion that they might not read well. They have often gotten along because of their intelligence, but have missed a lot because of poor reading and comprehension skills. These students often have decided that there is no hope or time for improvement. You may need to put some gentle pressure on such students to require them to seek help.

Once I asked one of my advisees who was failing a nursing class to show me how she read her assigned text. I found out that all she was reading were the first sentences of each paragraph and the content of tables and other figures. Although this technique might have been useful for a review, she was missing a lot of important information.

How Are the Student's Test-taking Skills?

Some students have difficulty taking tests, no matter how well prepared the students seem to be. If possible, get copies of tests the student has taken in the course in question. Go over items that were correctly as well as incorrectly answered, and ask the student to describe how each answer was selected. This will give you an idea of the student's thinking processes. Sometimes, she or he is reading too much into questions. You can help them to identify this problem and decrease its incidence by focusing only on each item's actual content.

Some students simply do not think through the question in a logical way. One student had missed an item on a nursing exam which concerned placement of pressure when withdrawing an intravenous needle. I asked her to describe to me what she thought when she was trying to answer that item. Instead of thinking about the positioning of the needle and her fingers *with a patient*, she had thought about doing it on her own arm. As a result, although she knew the right place to be applying pressure, she chose to answer "below the needle" instead of "above." I pointed out the error of thinking about procedures in the way she was.

Students who have severe test anxiety may need the assistance of a counselor or someone else specially prepared to assist students with such problems. You can offer some support for this, however. For example, find out if one particular aspect of the testing situation is causing difficulty. In most testing situations, students feel they have little control. It may help them if they can gain a sense of control through making decisions, such as selecting a specific place to sit. The student may need to enlist the instructor's assistance in such efforts. In many classes, students are assigned seating during tests and may not have much choice. The student and you may need to discuss this with the instructor to permit the student to have some autonomy within the teacher's parameters.

The best way to control test anxiety is for the student to be well prepared to take the test. This will be discussed in more detail later on.

How Are the Student's Writing Skills?

In some courses, part of the student's grade may be related to writing. Many college students have difficulty with this, no matter how hard the faculty in the English department try to help them learn the skills. I addressed ways of helping students to write in my previous book. Chapter 11 of this book should give you more ideas for helping students to write effectively.

Ask the student to let you read something she or he has written. Go over the paper and discuss ways of improving the most glaring problems. There are probably resources on your campus to help students improve their writing skills related to specific class requirements.

How Has the Student Been Studying for the Course?

Ask the student to describe their study methods. Some students do poorly because they have taken poor notes in the first place, or have not comprehended what they read. Therefore their study sessions based on these foundations are not productive. Once those problems are dealt with, the student's ability to study will be enhanced.

Many students benefit by studying with their classmates; weaker students may find this particularly helpful. Encourage your advisee to identify some of the stronger members of the class and negotiate with one or more of them to help in studying.

ADVISORY PROBLEMS

Adults require a different approach to academic advisement. Adult students such as RNs or students working on a second degree are often in as much need for support and guidance as the younger students. Many have been out of school for a long time, and they are unsure of negotiating the experience. However, what they may manifest is a false sense of assurance and a resistance to working with an advisor.

You need to convey to these adult advisees what you have to offer, and allow them to determine how they will comfortably work with you. I make sure my students know what things they will have to deal with me for, such as signing their registration forms, and I keep them well informed, so that they don't necessarily have to meet with me if they choose not to.

Even with all the effort I make to try to deal with adults on an adult level, many respond unexpectedly. Some feel that I have no time for them for the reasons given above: I don't require them to meet with me, and I make it possible for my students to get things accomplished without seeing me unnecessarily. They have difficulty being assertive enough to ask for more time when they want it.

On the other hand, some adult advisees feel that it's a direct affront to their competence that they are required to see me or contact me for anything. These folks are usually uncomfortable with being in the student role, and are resisting the feeling of dependence that the advisor-advisee relationship may imply. I try to reinforce their self-confidence and make it clear that I know they are capable of making their own decisions.

A lot of people seem to change their normal behavior when they assume the role of a student. Many of them are threatened by becoming a student again, and feel they will be treated like children. Ironically, they often behave in such a way that their prophecy becomes fulfilled. When this happens, it is important for you to continue to behave as one adult to the other until your advisee can resume a more appropriate level of functioning.

STUDENT ORGANIZATIONS

Students frequently require a consultant in organizational activities on and off-campus. This can be a very rewarding way in which to work with students outside the classroom. It can also be a challenge.

Students are often energetic and eager to be involved in organizations. They see it as a good way to make friends and to increase some of their skills. However, because of their youth and inexperience, they can sometimes make poor decisions which compromise the quality of their experience.

A faculty consultant can help students maximize their learning and minimize the risks of being active in an organization. The students are ultimately responsible for what happens with the organization, and the faculty consultant is only that: a consultant. A consultant in this context gives guidance, but students must make their own decisions. A faculty member who starts trying to run the organization or mold the leadership to her or his standards will compromise the integrity of the organization and undermine the students.

Before agreeing to be a consultant to an organization, make sure you understand the responsibilities this entails for you. Make sure you understand any liability you may be incurring by such a decision. Usually, as long as they are not minors, the elected officers of an organization have the fiduciary responsibility for the organization. This means that if they mismanage the organization and/or its funds, they can be held legally responsible. As a consultant, you need to be sure about your risk in such a case.

In addition to assessing your personal and financial liabilities, you need to become familiar with the following:

- bylaws of the organization;
- goals of the organization;
- organizational structure;
- history of the organization;
- current officers;

- level of participation of members;
- description of consultant's role;
- ties and interactions with other levels of the same organization; and
- relationships with other organizations

Listed below are some "Dos" and "Don'ts" for consultants.

DO:

- be available for reasonable amounts of consultation;
- help students to see more than one side of issues;
- help students to examine the risks and benefits of their decisions;
- give them guidelines instead of directions;
- talk to them as adults;
- allow them to make their own decisions;
- respect them;
- praise them for their work and their growth;
- help them to learn to find and use a variety of resources;
- help officers to learn to be available to members; and
- find ways for them to be rewarded and reinforced for giving organizational service.

DON'T:

- criticize them;
- second guess them;
- give them orders;
- minimize their efforts;
- ignore their concerns;
- let them get into financial trouble, if you can help them to avoid it;
- take on extra financial burdens yourself;
- start feeling the organization belongs to you; or
- talk to them like children or subordinates.

I served for several years as the school consultant or the consultant to a state nursing students' association. During that time, I always made it clear to the students and to others that I was their consultant, not their manager. I attended board meetings, state conventions, and accompanied my students to national conventions.

I must admit that at times it was very difficult to behave impartially when I had a bias about what was happening. You can, on occasion, offer advice, whether or not it is solicited. For example, if the group seems to be bogged down or floundering, or if the leaders seem to have difficulty figuring out what to do, you may need to be assertive about helping them to grapple with their responsibilities. On the other hand, even when the situation is at its worst, you must sometimes be patient enough to let the students figure out what they truly want to do, and give advice only when asked to do so. One of the most difficult times I ever experienced is described in Situation 5.1.

One of the most gratifying things about being a consultant to student organizations is watching students grow into leadership roles. Many of them have leadership traits before they ever run for office. They have developed these skills through previous experiences. Other students wait until they are in college to start venturing into these areas. Both types frequently need a consultant's support to carve out their own niche as a leader.

My style has always been to try to allow the students as much room as possible in which to function, unless they seem genuinely to be in trouble. I have frequently disagreed with decisions of the students I was advising, but I accorded them the respect they were due and kept my mouth shut unless asked for input. Generally, instead of telling them how I think they should deal with their difficulties, I refer them to their own organizational resources, such as their bylaws, policies, and other members.

Students may want their consultant to tell them what to do rather than simply give them advice. In addition, people outside the organization often think that the consultant should be telling the students what to do. Many of my colleagues have had the impression that the students did things because it was my idea and not their own. On the other hand, colleagues would sometimes tell me things they thought I should tell the students to do. I seemed always to be clarifying my role for someone. Situation 5.2 is a dramatic example of such an incident.

Another feature of consulting is traveling with the students to state or national conventions. I always felt it was important for me

Situation 5.1

Organization Consultant

Several years ago I was a consultant to the state nursing students association. At the first board meeting, the new president, Dan, took an adversarial role with the other officers, challenging them and asking why they hadn't started doing more. They were taken aback as was I, since this was their first meeting. After making everyone uncomfortable, Dan calmed down and started behaving more appropriately. When he gave us a break, the other consultant and I took him aside to offer some advice on better ways to deal with the other students. He was arrogant and stated he knew how to be president.

Over the next several months, Dan continued to harass the other board members while he did little to further the work of the group. All the board members, in contrast, worked diligently on planning for convention and other activities.

In the meantime, Dan was not doing well in school. Because of this he was unable to attend the national convention representing the state. However, he waited so long to let the vice president know of the situation that she was unable to attend in his place, and another officer had to serve as the state delegate.

Dan started missing meetings or canceling them at the last minute. The other officers were getting tired of his behavior and were worried about their plans, but they kept trying to work around him. Finally, he missed a meeting without calling anyone to explain his absence, and one of the other officers said, "We should impeach him."

Someone else asked if that was possible, and I told them to look at the bylaws. The bylaws provided for relieving an officer of her/his office if she/he failed to perform the duties of the office. The students asked me how this could be done.

I advised them to send Dan notice by registered mail that they had determined that he was not performing his duties. I told them to inform him that if he did not attend the next board meeting and explain what was happening, they would declare his office vacant. They voted to take this action and did so.

Dan did not come to the next meeting, nor did he notify the group that he would be absent. We waited a long time; one of the officers even tried calling Dan. It was hard for them to finally give up. They asked me how to make the motion, and I told them someone needed to move to declare the office of president vacant. One of them made the motion, which passed with no further discussion.

Throughout all this, I definitely wanted to see them divest themselves of this ineffective president, but I never suggested it. I waited for them to decide this was a move they wanted to make. Had they not decided to take that action, I would have advised them on how to proceed with an absent president.

Situation 5.2

Organization-Consultant Conflict

For many years, the nursing students' convention had been held in conjunction with the state nurses association (SNA) convention. Because of this, staff of the SNA did most of the work for the students while planning for their own convention.

One year, for several reasons, the students decided to hold their convention completely apart from SNA. I did not support their plan, and described some of the reasons I thought it was better for them to have their convention with the SNA. They listened but stuck to their decision. As faculty and officers of the SNA started finding out about this, I started hearing about it. These people seemed to think I could make the students do whatever I wanted. I explained my role, and pointed out that these students were adults. As adults, they had the right to run their organization as they saw fit. Some people from the SNA said I should not attend the student convention because it would look like I was supporting their decision. My response was essentially: "I *am* supporting their decision. They had a right to make it, and I won't abandon them for not taking my advice."

The student board was comprised of very strong people, some of whom were students at my school. They did an excellent job of planning for their convention. Shortly before the convention date, the president of the National Student Nurses Association (NSNA) called the state president and said she would be attending the convention. We were delighted.

When the NSNA president arrived, she was rather cool toward me. This surprised me, because she and I had talked many times and had always had a warm relationship. The second day of the convention, two of the officers asked me to meet with them and the NSNA president. The president had already talked to the students about most of what she proceeded to tell me: that she had come to our convention because two people from the SNA had contacted the national office. They had reported that I was interfering with the students and that I was the one who got them to break away from holding simultaneous conventions with the SNA. The NSNA president had discussed this with the officers who set her straight immediately and who wanted her to talk to me.

Then the NSNA president told us all something she hadn't told the others first. In order to make this appearance, and try what she had thought was damage control, she had canceled a special trip to an international meeting in Europe which was to have been followed by a

Continued on next page

visit to the ICN Headquarters. We were speechless at first; then all four of us had tears rolling down our cheeks.

I will never forget the scene: the four of us sitting there, trying to take in the fact that we had been manipulated by someone who was actually doing what I had been accused of doing. We formed a bond; I am still in touch with all the others. The officers took up a collection among themselves to buy the NSNA president a brass hourglass which they presented to her at the closing session. She helped to install the new officers, and by the time the meeting broke up, almost all of us were crying from the emotional strain.

Although it was a stressful experience, we all learned far more from it than if we had done what we were *supposed* to do. I think it also showed us how important it is to do the right thing. Sometimes the right thing may not be what you want to do, but it is right, nonetheless. The students did the right thing, by asserting their independence. I did the right thing by fulfilling my duties as their consultant. The NSNA president did the right thing by coming to help when she thought it was warranted. It was one of those situations that seemed bad at first, but turned into something very special. All of those of us who were aware of what was happening behind the scenes were changed by the experience.

to be warm and friendly to the students, yet to maintain my role as a consultant. This meant keeping a bit of distance in some situations so that I was not compromised and yet was available for assistance.

Since these were college students of legal age, paying their own expenses, I had no responsibility for enforcing any particular standards of behavior. As long as the students weren't doing anything dangerous or illegal, I usually kept my mouth shut. Sometimes their behavior could be outrageous, and sometimes deliberately so in order to see if they could get a reaction from me and other consultants. As in most such cases, the best way to deal with it is to ignore it.

One thing which I felt indicated my accessibility and appeal for students as their consultant was that it was sometimes difficult to have any time away from them at meetings. My students wanted me to sit with them, visit their bull sessions after meetings, attend all the social events, eat with them, and generally be with them most of the time. When I was younger and could still keep up, I enjoyed being included in these activities. As I attended more and more of these meetings, I tried to impose more distance between us. With some groups, this was relatively easy. However, some students were more interested than others in opportunities to get to know the consultants more informally.

SOCIALIZING WITH STUDENTS

Whether you are an academic advisor, organizational consultant, or have any other contacts outside the classroom, you need to be wise about how you interact with students. You must be aware not only of what you do and say, but also of how your behavior appears to others. Keep the following points in mind:

Unless your students are truly underage, *don't take on the parental role*. Treat them like the adults they are.

Be yourself and be comfortable at social events.

If you don't approve of a particular behavior, *voice your concerns*, but don't try to enforce change which is not in your field of control over the student.

Don't reveal intimate information about your life or about your family. It's fine to share general information about your marital status, and about your spouse and/or children, but do not confide too much in students.

Don't be alone with a student in a situation which could lead to confusion about role boundaries and your behavior.

Don't get involved in a sexual relationship with a student while he or she is a student and you're a faculty member.

Don't tell students personal things about other faculty members.

Don't talk to students about intra-faculty conflicts and problems.

Avoid situations in which you are pitted with the students against other faculty members.

CONCLUSION

One of the rewards of being a faculty member is being able to work with students in a variety of ways outside the classroom. As long as your responsibilities and privileges in these situations are clear, these associations should be a satisfying addition to your total experience of working with students.

SIX

Planning and Implementing Your Professional Development Plan

• •

A faculty member not only needs to but wants to continue to develop professionally. Some states have specific requirements for you, as a registered nurse, to participate in a certain number of hours of continuing education appropriate to your practice. To get the most out of your activities, it will help you to plan for both short-term and long-term goals.

PURPOSE

The purpose of this chapter is to help you to identify and engage in appropriate activities to maintain and extend your professional expertise.

PLANNING

You should have a general plan for your ongoing professional development. This doesn't need to be terribly formal, and it should be flexible enough to adjust both to changes in your schedule and unexpected opportunities. Table 6.1 gives an example of a professional development plan.

If you set objectives, your planned activities will be more obvious. You should include not only workshops and the like, but also reading you plan to accomplish. Once you have identified the activities in which you might participate, you should establish your priorities.

Although you should arrange for the time and money to do these things, you may receive some help from your school. Goals and a structured plan may help you make a case for financial assistance. Although many schools limit their assistance to support of major presentations at prestigious meetings, others have some funding available to assist faculty members who need it. The bottom line, though, is that you are responsible for your own development.

PROFESSIONAL MEETINGS

Some events occur on a regular basis, and you know well in advance whether or not they will fit into your plans. For example, your state nurses association has a convention every year. Your district nurses association has regularly scheduled meetings. If you are a member of Sigma Theta Tau, you can attend regularly scheduled meetings, often focusing on research. In the fall of odd-numbered years, Sigma Theta Tau holds an international convention; in the alternate years, there are Regional Assemblies.

The American Nurses Association holds its national conventions in the summer of even-numbered years. The National League for Nursing holds conventions in the summer of odd-numbered years. If you are in a specialty organization, you may already know or can easily find out when local, regional, and national meetings will be held.

Nursing journals usually carry notices of many types of workshops and other programs. Of course, you are most likely to find what you are looking for in a journal that is directly related to your interests. If you are interested in a certain focus in research, calls for abstracts often precede formal announcements of meetings by several months. However, whether you plan to submit an

Table 6.1

Professional Development Plan

PROFESSIONAL DEVELOPMENT PLAN
1992 – 1993
OBJECTIVES

1. Maintain my general knowledge of the nursing profession.
2. Continue to increase my expertise in working with children, especially dying children.
3. Improve my test construction abilities.
4. Increase my knowledge of the use of qualitative research methodology.

ACTIONS

GENERAL

FNA Convention programs, September (2 – 3 Contact Hours (CHs))*
FNA Disaster Nursing workshop, Orlando, March (6 CHs)

CLINICAL

FNA Council on Child Health, Orlando, September (1 CH)*
FNA Council on Bioethics, Orlando, September (1 CH)*
Symposium on dying children, St. Louis, November (6 CHs)

TEACHING

Work with Dr. Mathis on test construction, Fall*

RESEARCH

Sigma Theta Tau Research Day, October (5 CHs)
Read each issue of *Nursing Research*
Read book on qualitative methodology, October – January*

---

*My priorities

abstract or not, this will give you enough notice to plan on attending, if you are interested in the content.

Many groups mail calls for abstracts and meeting notices to nurses on selected mailing lists, as well as to schools of nursing in the particular region. Most schools have a central place where this information can be found, such as a bulletin board in a faculty area. If there isn't such a service, you might suggest that one be started, or volunteer to start and maintain it if the information is forwarded to you.

Another way to find out about things that might interest you is to talk to your colleagues about your specific interests. Ask them to let you know if they happen to hear of something in your area. By the same token, you should be willing to do the same to help them.

If you are interested in continuing education by home study, and if continuing education is mandated in your state, you won't have to worry about getting information. People offering continuing education will find you. Alternatively, you can get in touch with these groups and ask to be placed on their mailing lists.

ADVANCED DEGREES

If you want to work on your doctorate, you also need a plan. Decide when and where you will do it. Many nursing faculty members work on their doctorates while they continue to teach. This means they either have to live near a doctoral program where they can continue in their teaching position, or they have to move to a new area where they can find both a teaching position and a suitable program.

Either of the above options requires planning. You need to learn about the doctoral programs available in the area of study that interests you. You must establish the parameters which will determine your choice. The process begins by asking yourself questions about what you want.

What Field Do You Want Your Doctorate In?

Actually, some people make this choice after answering the next question. Ideally, your choice includes nursing, education, or related fields. You need to consider this carefully because it will determine what you can do for the rest of your career. For example, some nursing schools already have a preference for faculty members with doctorates in nursing. Schools with high prestige, where there is considerable competition for faculty positions, might be less interested in you, regardless of your other strengths, if you don't hold this doctorate.

Your career goals should determine what field you study. Talk with seasoned faculty members who have a national perspective about their perceptions of the relevance of a given degree to the way you see yourself functioning in the future.

Are You Willing and Able To Relocate?

If you can and would relocate, are there any limits about where you would go? Some people are willing to stay in their current region; others want to go to only specific parts of the country. This is one way to establish the field of possibilities.

Once you've answered the above questions, you're ready to consider the options. Then you can plan for achieving the goals you set.

Establish Your Criteria for Selection

You need to decide what is important to you about the place you attend. Even while you are still identifying programs, this will help you to get more information. However, don't rule out some schools too early just because you know or have heard little about them. While they may have very good quality programs, their profile might be lower than other schools.

Some of the factors you might consider in selecting a school would include:

- Competition to get accepted;
- Cost of tuition and cost of living;
- Employment opportunities;
- Faculty;
- Location (e.g., small town or large city);
- Program components;
- Reputation of the university and the specific program in which you are interested;
- Requirements for students;

- Research opportunities for graduate students; and
- Research in progress by faculty.

Identify appropriate programs

You can get lists of doctoral programs in nursing through many sources. The National League for Nursing and the American Association of Colleges of Nursing has such lists available upon request. If you are choosing another field of study, you might start by identifying the universities in the geographic areas you are looking at. Any large university is likely to have the program you want in such fields as education, psychology, or public health.

One way of finding programs in fields outside of nursing is to look in the relevant professional journals. If they carry announcements of available faculty positions, you can identify some possibilities. When you're looking at journal articles, see if you find information about the schools where authors attended or where they appear to be teaching. *The Chronicle of Higher Education* often contains articles about specific programs, as well as other announcements which may give you leads.

Getting information

Write or call the schools which sound promising and request university catalogs and information about the specific program in which you're interested.

Evaluating the possibilities

Once you have the information, you can use your criteria to determine which schools are truly likely possibilities. Talk to people you respect to find out if they know about the universities and schools you're considering. Once you start narrowing down your choices, you might want to consider visiting the likely prospects. If possible, request an interview with someone who can talk with you about the program. If you get such an interview, go prepared with a list of questions and concerns to discuss.

Apply for your top choices

You need to decide if your priority is to get started in a doctoral program at a particular time, or to wait until you are accepted into a particular program. If you are determined to start at a particular time, you may have to settle for your second or third choice. If you are willing to wait to be accepted by a particular program, make sure you have a chance of eventually being accepted.

CONCLUSION

As with any activity, the only way to accomplish a goal is to make sure you know what your goal is and to make a plan to achieve it. Whether or not you have finished your formal education, you need to plan for attendance at professional meetings. If you still need to earn your doctorate, you must approach that phase of your education in an organized way.

Developing Your Research Program

· ·

Most faculty members are expected to be involved to some degree in conducting research. The requirements for your level of activity will vary throughout your career. Your activity will also be determined by other factors, such as the nature of the institution. For example, some universities are research-oriented as a primary function. The expectation for you to conduct, complete, and publish research will be greater in such places than at smaller liberal arts universities.

Wherever you are working, you need to verify what the expectations are. If you plan to remain on the faculty and seek continued employment, you need to know how the presence or absence of research will affect your status. In many institutions, published research is a *minimum* expectation for any kind of advance in rank or for retention within the tenure system.

You will be best able to conduct, complete, and publish research if you have a plan for doing so. Too many faculty members wander aimlessly through their careers without making a plan, and thus never achieve much in the way of results. The sooner you develop your plan and start implementing it, the more effective you will be.

87

PURPOSES

The purposes of this chapter are to help you to:

- choose a research focus;
- formulate a research activity plan;
- make time to conduct research;
- find resources to help you in conducting research; and
- collaborate with others to produce research.

CHOOSING A RESEARCH FOCUS

As nursing matures as a discipline, research activities in graduate education are also changing. Many people are studying significant issues for their thesis level of research. Ideally this should form the foundation of future research activities, both in and out of a doctoral program. However, some people become interested in new things once they have completed their MSNs (or doctorates).

The most important thing is to identify an area to which to direct your attention. If you have many and diverse interests, this may seem to be a difficult task. However, most of us can't study everything we're interested in, so we have to narrow it down in some way.

If you look at the most successful researchers who present and publish consistently and who are able to get funding, you will see that they are very focused in their activities. They have chosen to concentrate on a particular area, and their activities have built upon one another.

You may target a very specific area of study, such as the coping skills of new parents. In this event, you focus more and more in depth on this issue. On the other hand, you might target the broader area of interest, which is coping skills. Then you might work on expanding the concept in broadening perspectives on coping skills when describing a variety of populations or situations.

These are some questions you can ask yourself which may help you to discriminate what you're most interested in studying.

Is One Area Understudied?

If you can identify an area in which not much work is going on, your efforts may receive more notice.

Does the Nursing Model to Which You Subscribe Indicate An Area For Study?

If something you are interested in fits well within a theoretical framework, you will find it easier to design studies around it.

Is One Area Related Specifically to Content You Plan to Teach?

Expanding your investigations around things you teach will add to your expertise.

Is One Area More Likely Than Others to be Funded by Grants?

Even if you are doing preliminary research, choosing an area likely to be supported in the future will give you a track record which will improve your chances of garnering such funding.

Which Topic Is Sufficiently Interesting to Make You Want to Study It for a Part of Your Career?

If you are going to live with this topic for a few years, or even the rest of your career, you want to pick something stimulating which will sustain your interest.

Is There a Potential Co-investigator Or Group With Whom You Want to Work?

If you have one or more colleagues who are interested, you may select a topic of mutual interest.

You may come up with other questions which are more pertinent to you and your interests. However, the most important principle is not to waste your energies by choosing nothing or by not getting started on the project you've chosen.

FORMULATING A RESEARCH PLAN

You may take a while to decide where you want to invest your research energy, but you need to choose something within your first year as a faculty member. You may reconsider and change your focus later, but you must decide during that first year; or you probably will not complete anything.

You should plan not only for the current study but also for further studies and project their likely timetables. If you project future research in this way, you will be in a better position to implement them later. For example, by planning for the future, you will have something to move right into while previous studies are being reviewed for publication.

A sample research program plan is shown in Table 7.1. As you can see, it is fairly general. Once you are dealing with a specific study, you would have more exact timelines. Once a researcher becomes productive, she or he will often do some work on the next study while still involved with the first.

Start out with a simple plan for the first one or two studies. As you become more experienced, you will learn what you can expect of yourself given the requirements of your teaching position and the demands of your personal life.

MAKING TIME FOR RESEARCH

If you hope that opportunities to do research will present themselves without your looking for them, you will probably be disappointed. An educator's busy schedule can manage to take up all your time. The only way to *get* time to do research is to *make* time for it.

We all know we have only 24 hours in the day. You can't really "make" time. However, you can organize your time so that you will be able to accomplish the priorities you set. Once you determine that working on your research is a priority, you must establish parameters for yourself to be successful. Some suggestions are described below, and are also listed in Table 7.2.

With research, as with your other projects, you will probably find it helpful to work on a regular basis. This will work best if you spend time with it at least once a week. Even if all you are doing is looking up references or organizing what you already have, this will keep you involved and keep your momentum going.

Establish specific times to work. For example, you may dedicate every Friday afternoon to your research. Mark this on your calendar to make sure you do not schedule anything else in that time. If conflicts arise, set a specific alternate time during the week to make up for any regular time you miss.

At some points in working on a study, you will need more time than the block you have set aside. When that happens, set more specific times to do specific work, such as assembling packets for

Table 7.1

Research Program Plan

FOCUS: STRESS MASTERY IN DYING CHILDREN

Time lines   Activities

STUDY #1
9/93 – 12/93 Literature review
                                        Tool review and selection
1/94 – 3/94   Write proposal for initial study
3/94 – 6/94   Collect data
7/94 – 9/94   Analyze data and write results
10/94   Submit manuscript for publication
10/94 – 95   Revise manuscript if requested and/or
                                        submit to other journals

STUDY #2
11/94 – 2/95 Update literature review
3/95 – 5/95   Write proposal focusing on new aspects
                                        indicated by Study #1
5/95 – 9/95   Collect and analyze data; write results
10/95   Submit manuscript for publication
10/95 – 96   Revise manuscript if requested and/or
                                        submit to other journals

STUDY #3   Instrument Design
5/95 – 10/95 Identify funding resources for Study #3
                                        Get application materials, etc., to apply for
                                        funding
11/95 – 4/96 Write proposal for Study #3 to design an
                                        instrument
                                        Apply for funding of Study #3
?/96 – ?/97   Conduct study within parameters relevant
                                        to funding
?/97   Complete reports required by funding
                                        agency
                                        Submit manuscript for publication

Study #4 and future studies: Timelines to be determined

Table 7.2

Managing Time to Do Research

Set aside a specific time each week to work on your research. For example: Every Friday from 1–4; Tuesday from 3–6 and Thursday from 9–12.

If you have to miss your regularly scheduled time, set another time to make up for it.

When you have more to do than usual, add time to work on your research each week, rather than spreading it out over several weeks.

If you feel you need a break from your research, set specific parameters for yourself. For example: How long a break are you going to take? (2 weeks, a month?); establish exactly when you will resume your work (On March 30; the second week of the semester).

When you're having trouble staying focused, don't quit working altogether. You may spend less time per day, but do something every day at the regular time.

When you are in a writing phase, write something every day of the week.

When there is a lag in your current research, do some work for the next one.

participants or analyzing results. Often these are activities about which you will be enthused, and you won't find it as difficult to work as when things are going more slowly.

At some times, you may come to a point where you feel you need a break from your research, or other demands on your time may require you to stop working for a while. When this happens, set specific boundaries for your break. Establish how long you will be away from your research and the specific time when you will resume your work. Write these deadlines down on your calendar. The more you formalize it, the more useful the break will be and the more likely it will be that you will resume when you really mean to do so.

Sometimes it may be hard to stay focused and keep working, such as when you are in the phase of writing the proposal or the final manuscript. At these times, you should work on your project *more* frequently, and not *less* frequently, than usual. Make yourself do something every day, even if it's simply fixing the margins on the document, or reorganizing your notes. If you spend too much time away from your project, you're setting yourself up for failure.

One of the advantages of having a long-term plan is that you may be able to do some work toward an upcoming study during lag times of your current one. Sometimes, when you feel you can't look at the current project for one more minute, shifting your focus to the future research that will result will give you the boost you need to complete the work.

FINDING RESOURCES

To find adequate resources, you need to identify what you need for the study you plan to conduct. Start by working out a budget and by listing the nonfinancial support you need.

BUDGET

In beginning studies which will receive minimal funding, you will probably not find enough financial support to pay for your time spent on the research. However, you should still calculate the cost of this time. If you are able to negotiate for this as part of your faculty contract, at least it will be accounted for.

Table 7.3 lists some of the items to consider including in your budget. Not every study will require each of these items. The cost of some things may be negligible because you already have the resources, for example, storage of materials relating to your study. Be aware that this list is not exhaustive, your study may have some special financial requirements.

A budget will help you to be realistic about your planning and may make you aware of factors which necessitate modifications of your plans. Even if you think the costs will be minimal, you should have a budget written down. This will be a fundamental expectation of funding agencies, even if you apply for only seed money.

Table 7.3

Items for a Budget

Your time
Data collectors' time
Purchase price of printed instruments
Equipment and nonprinted instruments
Printing
Photocopying
Secretarial time
Literature search
Travel
Office space
    Work space
    Interview room
    Furniture
Supplies
    Paper
    Envelopes
    Stationery
    Pencils
    Audiotapes
    Computer disks
Computer/word processor
Postage
Telephone
    Basic
    Long distance
Payment for subjects
Data analysis
    Statistician
    Computer time
Storage

PEOPLE

If research is an expectation within your institution, there probably are some systems built in to support it. There may be a unit dedicated to research support within your school or within the university. This person or these people can provide a variety of assistance. Find out if such a unit exists. Then find out what their designated responsibilities are and how you might take advantage of their services.

Depending on the role such individuals are asked to fill, you may get anything from a little to a lot of support. Sometimes, these people can help even the novice researcher get started with a research study. Others are more dedicated to helping advanced investigators in getting large amounts of funding. Even if they have limited time to spend with novices, these people can probably help you if you have specific questions.

There are usually more experienced researchers on the faculty. Talk with them about their activities and how they organize themselves. You will find that there are many ways to conduct productive research.

ADMINISTRATIVE SUPPORT

As you design your research plan, you need to start identifying the types of support you will need. When you are negotiating for your work load, be sure to build in your need for time to do your research. This should be documented in some way, ideally as part of your formal contract.

You should also negotiate for other forms of help in addition to requesting the time. A novice researcher will have difficulty getting funding apart from small grants of around $500 to $1000. This rarely makes a dent in ambitious plans that require secretarial services, postage, and robust data analysis. Some of these needs may be met within the institution. For example, you may get permission to ask the secretary who regularly does typing for you to work on this as well. You may be permitted to use the school's bulk mail stamp to send out mailed surveys. When you make these arrangements, put them in writing and have them verified by the administrator concerned. This will help to prevent embarrassing misunderstandings.

GRANTS

There are many resources available to instruct you on grant applications. The NIH Guide is available from the U.S. Department of Health and Human Services. This guide lists calls for grants and contracts and specifies requirements for their application. Wilson (1989) has excellent information on writing proposals, as do other research texts. What I'm going to include here will be the barest minimum.

When you are applying for a grant, each funding source will have a particular format for your application, and some will have specific forms which you must complete. Therefore, your first step is to get this procedural information. After that, the overriding principle is for you to follow the format or submit the form exactly as specified. In some funding situations, there is so much competition that your application will be discarded if you fail to comply with the application requirements.

In general, proposals or applications for funding will follow the standard format for proposals. However, you will need to tailor your proposal to the specific goals of the funding source. Write your proposal carefully and have it reviewed by one or more colleagues with expertise in getting funding. Ask to look at proposals submitted by colleagues who have received funding. This will help you to identify the characteristics of success.

Give your proposal an effective *title*, as short as possible and understandable to the people who will review it. In other words, if reviewers will be from disciplines other than nursing, don't use language in the title that they wouldn't recognize, such as the names of nurse theorists.

Include an *introduction* or *summary* of four or five well-chosen statements which will stimulate interest and encourage further reading. Document the *need* for the study and link that to the purposes of the funding organization itself. Give a brief overview of the research with attention to how your proposed study will illuminate or expand what has already been done. Describe how the *outcomes* of your study will improve the lives of the kind of people you are studying. Describe or include *support* you will receive from relevant sources, such as institutions or individuals relevant to the study. Describe your plans for *publishing* the results.

Throughout your proposal, use logical lines of thought. Back up any claims or statistics with good references. If you think there will be any doubts about such references, attach copies of the supporting literature, if possible. Describe your experience as a researcher and do your best to show your capability to conduct your study.

WORKING WITH A TEAM

There are many benefits to working with colleagues in conducting research. The principal one is that with more minds involved, some issues will be better considered than if only one person was working on them. You may have a greater variety of strengths and talents than if you were working alone. As part of a team, novice researchers can work with more seasoned investigators and add to their knowledge and skills, while someone else may take on the brunt of the more technical concerns. Finally, the work can be distributed among several people so that you can get more done faster, or so that you may be able to do a more complex study.

Usually, it is best if one person is designated as the *principal investigator*. This person will coordinate the activities of the group, arrange for meetings, follow up on assignments, and take the lead in those writing activities which are part of the project. The principal investigator will usually be the most experienced member of the group, although at times it may be someone else due to that experienced person's other responsibilities.

When your group begins collaborating, you may want to set down some *ground rules* which will guide your work together. For example, you may want to specify how frequently you will meet. Identify the method you will use to surmount differences of opinion. Some of the guidelines given in Chapter 8 concerning working on committees may help you to handle such problems.

Whenever you do meet with your co-investigators, keep *notes* of the meetings. These don't have to be very formal, but one person should be designated to take them each time. After the meetings, these notes should be typed and distributed to all the members of the group. This will help to avoid problems caused by misunderstandings and untested assumptions.

Whether you are working with one co-investigator or with a group, your group may want to draw up an *agreement* concerning

Table 7.4

Agreement for a Group of Investigators

STUDY: STRESS MASTERY IN CHILDREN WITH CANCER

PRINCIPAL INVESTIGATOR: MARY LOWE

CO-INVESTIGATORS: MARTHA GILBERT, LOUISE MILLBURN, TOM SANFORD

POINTS OF AGREEMENT

1. Mary Lowe will be the principal investigator. She will:
   chair meetings of the group;
   verify that the other investigators have completed their assignments;
   maintain any files related to the study; and
   be the first name listed on any publications or other information about this study.
2. All members will participate equally in all other aspects of the study:
   taking notes of meetings;
   writing the proposal;
   collecting data;
   analyzing data;
   writing the manuscript for publication; and
   making presentations.
   Co-investigators' names will always be listed alphabetically.
3. Major decisions about the study will be arrived at by unanimous consent before work proceeds.
4. As far as possible, decisions will be reached through group discussion and will be accepted unanimously.
5. If agreement cannot be reached on a substantive issue, the group will work toward trying to achieve agreement, through continued discussion, more investigation, or consultation with others.
6. If agreement cannot be reached on nonsubstantive issues, decisions will be made by the majority.
7. Publications and presentations will always be done by the entire group, unless one member is unable to participate or if it is impractical in the context.

your individual and group responsibilities. This will help to clarify from the outset who is in charge of what and what time commitments are expected of all participants. A sample of such a contract is in Table 7.4. Your study or the mix of people involved may warrant different components, but this will give you an idea of some of the factors which you will need to consider.

CONCLUSION

The key to a successful research program is planning. A well-considered plan enhances your chances of producing meaningful results. You must be well-organized and develop realistic time frames within which to work. If you collaborate with others in conducting a study, organization and a certain degree of formality in your procedures will contribute to a harmonious and productive relationship with your colleagues.

REFERENCES

Selby, M. L., Riportella-Muller, R., & Farel, A. (1992). Building administrative support for your research: A neglected key for turning a research plan into a funded project. *Nursing Outlook, 40,* 73–77.

Wilson, H. (1989). *Research in Nursing.* Redwood City, CA: Addison-Wesley.

············ EIGHT ············

Working on Committees

Committees are a fact of life in most large organizations, and especially typical of academic settings. Committees are groups of people who are responsible for accomplishing designated tasks. Some groups are simply responsible for regularly occurring tasks; which are important for the smooth functioning of an organization; these committees have little status or prestige attached to membership. Others are responsible for such significant activities that their membership carries special privileges or status. Over your years as a faculty member, you will have the opportunity to serve on both types of committees, with opportunities for the second emerging after you have achieved other marks of accomplishment or longevity.

PURPOSES

This chapter will help you to:

- identify the roles of committees;
- choose committees on which to serve;
- function effectively as a committee member;
- take appropriate meeting minutes; and
- serve as an effective chairperson of a committee.

101

COMMITTEES

Following is a discussion of some committees which are typical in schools of nursing and the universities of which they are a part. Their usual functions are briefly described here; refer to the appropriate publications within your school for information about specific tasks. Some of these groups may have different designations than "committee" in your situation, but their functions will be similar.

Before examining the various committees and their responsibilities, understand the two important considerations that pertain to any committee or similar group. First, *extent and limits of authority* of the committee should always be clear. Some committees make policy; others merely recommend policies. Some committees may determine the actions they will take, while others carry out actions assigned to them by others.

The other important consideration is *to whom the committee is responsible*. Some committees report to the faculty as a whole; any actions they recommend cannot be undertaken without approval from the total faculty. Other committees will be responsible to the dean or some other administrator. Whenever you work on a committee, you must be clear on these lines of authority so that you do not exceed your responsibility.

STRUCTURAL COMMITTEES

Structural committees constitute the working groups of the organization's structure. Faculty are usually members without regard to their specific positions within the school, and either volunteer or are appointed from the general faculty. Some may be there in an *ex officio* capacity.

Some committees require that their members fit a particular description, such as being tenured or holding a minimum faculty rank. Such committees usually have prestige because of the membership requirements.

Committees are usually described and their functions and membership specified in faculty bylaws or other similar documents that describe the structure of the school or university. This should be the final reference for you in reviewing your institutional structure.

Committees can be broadly classified as concerning *academic affairs, faculty affairs,* and *student affairs.* In a small school with few faculty members, there might be only committees with these three designations. They would do all the work within each broad area, perhaps breaking into subcommittees for occasional intensive tasks. In a larger school, different, separate committees might focus on some specific areas of concern.

Academic Affairs

These committees deal with concerns such as:

- developing, evaluating, and revising curriculum;
- evaluating the program and its resources;
- developing policies on grading and evaluation of students; and
- monitoring learning resources such as library and computer support.

Faculty Affairs

The responsibilities of these committees include:

- searching for, recruiting, interviewing, and advising the dean on hiring prospective faculty members;
- orienting new faculty members;
- overseeing the policies and processes in the evaluation and progression of faculty;
- reviewing and recommending action on faculty applying for continuing contracts or tenure;
- developing and revising faculty position descriptions;
- developing policies about and monitoring faculty workload;
- overseeing faculty benefits and welfare;
- organizing and coordinating faculty development activities;
- establishing and implementing mechanisms for the recognition and reward of faculty accomplishments;
- reviewing requests for institutional grants, leaves, and sabbaticals;
- reviewing research proposals;
- developing policies for and implementing faculty grievance procedures;

- reviewing and recommending amendments to faculty by-laws;
- providing a handbook of faculty policies; and
- planning and implementing faculty activities such as agency recognition events, newsletters, and faculty social events.

Student Affairs

These committees may be responsible for some of the activities outlined under "Academic Affairs" which directly involve students. They might also be responsible for:

- developing policies for and overseeing the recruitment, admission, retention, progression, dismissal, and graduation of students;
- developing policies for and responding to student appeals or grievances related to grades and other issues;
- facilitating access of students to financial aid;
- developing and updating student policy manuals;
- establishing and coordinating recognitions for student achievements; and
- organizing and coordinating student activities such as clubs and ceremonial events.

ADMINISTRATIVE COMMITTEES

There are two types of administrative committees. The first is a representative body composed partly or completely of elected faculty members. On a university level, this would include the *faculty senate*: elected faculty members who represent their respective schools. Administrators may attend these committee meetings with or without a voice, but usually without a vote. On the school level, a similar group might be called the *faculty board* or *faculty executive committee*. Members would include the faculty secretary and treasurer as well as representatives of groups within the school. Administrators such as the dean and associate or assistant deans are likely to serve on these committees with both voice and vote.

These groups make policies, oversee their implementation, and evaluate outcomes. They sometimes serve as the ad hoc by-laws committee for the larger organization.

The second type of administrative committee is the *executive committee* or *administrative council* for the school or university. This would include the administrators of the level such as the school. These groups deal with administrative concerns in running the university or school.

Another administrative committee is the advisory council to administrators. The members of such a committee are selected by the administrator. These groups would discuss concerns affecting the administrative purview. However, as advisory bodies, they take no action that extends beyond their group. On the other hand, the administrator may develop or implement new approaches based on the committee's recommendations.

COMMITTEE MEMBER ROLES

CHAIRPERSON

The *chairperson* of a structural committee may be appointed by a higher authority, such as the administrator or the administrative committee to which the committee reports. Sometimes the chairperson is elected by the committee's own members. For faculty administrative committees, the dean or director may serve as the chairperson, or the chairperson may be elected from the faculty. Usually, the senior administrator serves as chair of the other administrative committees mentioned.

The chairperson is responsible for preparing for meetings. Usually, the chairperson develops the *agenda* for each meeting. This agenda is fairly general and may include the names of the individuals who are responsible for each topic. The agenda may be distributed to members as a way of reminding them of the meeting and of the business to be conducted, or it can be distributed at the meeting. A sample agenda appears in Table 8.1.

The agenda gives the committee members an idea of what will happen at the meeting. It also enables them to bring the materials necessary to participate, such as the position descriptions to be discussed, or the faculty handbook.

Depending on the situation, the chairperson may or may not be responsible for *notifying members* of the meeting times. In some institutions, the meeting days and times are determined at the beginning of the year, and may always be held on the same day of

Table 8.1

Meeting Agenda

ALPHA BETA SCHOOL OF NURSING
FACULTY AFFAIRS COMMITTEE
AGENDA

DATE AND TIME	February 11, 1993, 10:00 AM	
PLACE	Conference Room, 3rd floor	
CALL TO ORDER		A. Miller, Chair
MINUTES		M. Pauley
OLD BUSINESS		
	Agency Workshop	D. Duncan
	Search Subcommittee	S. Taylor
	Updates for Handbook	A. Miller
NEW BUSINESS		
	Position Descriptions	A. Miller
	Social Affairs	M. Pauley
	Other Business	
NEXT MEETING	March 11, 1993	
ADJOURNMENT		

the month at the same time. Under such circumstances, the chairperson may not feel the need to send out reminders. However, if meetings are scheduled less regularly, a reminder may help to ensure that all members will be present.

The chairperson may be responsible for making other *arrangements*, such as reserving the meeting room, unless that is assigned by another authority. If committee members require printed materials to adequately participate, the chairperson should see that these materials are duplicated and distributed either in advance or at the meeting.

The chairperson *presides* at each meeting. This includes calling the meeting to order and seeing that the business proceeds in a timely fashion. Although many procedures relevant to large groups are also applicable to committees, there are some exceptions. The chairperson of a committee is expected to be a working member and an active participant in discussions. The chairperson has a vote along with the other members, not only in the event of a tie. Whether the group is large or small, the idea of rules of order is to maintain order and see that the rights of the minority as well as of the majority are protected (Robert, 1967). The chairperson determines when the meeting should adjourn and verifies that all members understand what they are responsible to accomplish before the next meeting. Many people who serve as chairperson like to review the meeting minutes for accuracy before they are circulated.

SECRETARY

The *secretary*, or recorder, is responsible for accurately recording the actions of the committee. The secretary makes sure that the minutes are typed and properly distributed. The latter process usually includes ensuring that a copy of the minutes is placed in a specified file or notebook. The secretary should find out if the chairperson wants to review the minutes before they are distributed. (The details of this process are described in a later section.)

MEMBERS

Although the chairperson and the secretary participate as members, there are other *members* who may not have such designated responsibilities. Most members serve either as members at large, representing no one group, or as representatives of certain groups, such as the graduate or undergraduate faculty.

Other people may serve as ex officio members. An *ex officio member* is one who serves by virtue of holding a particular office or position. For example, the dean may be an ex officio member of all standing committees in the school of nursing. According to Robert (1967), an ex officio member has all the rights and privileges of any other member, including voting, unless these rights are limited in the rules or bylaws of the group. However, the ex officio member has none of the obligations of other members. This means that an ex officio member is not required to attend meetings, or to serve as the secretary or chairperson of the committee.

A member is responsible for arriving at the meeting both on time and prepared for the discussion as indicated in the agenda. If a member must be absent, it is courteous of them to inform the chairperson ahead of the meeting time. During a meeting, each member should participate in the discussion and help in arriving at consensus, if that is the style of the committee.

Each member should share the duties for which the committee is responsible. Novices may have time to become accustomed to the committee's work. However, those members who have experience in other committees may be able to begin participating quickly because of their familiarity with committee work in general. Virtually everyone on a faculty committee has many responsibilities of their own. Regardless of how busy you feel you are, you should take your turn in fulfilling the obligations of the committee.

Members with an assignment to complete outside the meeting should be prepared to inform the chairperson and the other committee members of their progress. Members who have completed these assignments may need to submit written or oral reports of their work. The format will usually be determined by the structure of the institution, or by the chairperson.

DECISION MAKING BY CONSENSUS

Many groups within work settings function not on the basis of "majority rule," but by consensus seeking. Motions may be made in either system. A motion made in a committee does not require a second, and members are not required to stand while speaking, unless the committee is large (Robert, 1967). After the motion is made, the manner of proceeding will differ according to the accepted mode of decision making in the committee. If the majority will determine the outcome, a vote is taken at the end of discussion, and the disposition of the question is determined by the vote of the majority. If there is to be a decision by consensus, the discussion proceeds, if possible, until all members agree. A statement of consensus should be made by the chair and recorded just as a vote would be.

Consensus is a term used to connote general agreement, and usually unanimity. It is different from *compromise*, in which all the parties involved have to give up something. In consensus, the emphasis is on all parties finding a mutually designed solution in which they all can feel they have won. Nichols (1982) noted the pervasive use of voting and majority rule in academic communities. Nichols pointed out that majority voting tends to leave a dissatisfied minority and engenders a climate which does not encourage people to express their best ideas.

EXPECTING CONSENSUS

One important factor in encouraging consensus is the *expectation* of it. The person in charge should be clear that this will be the decision-making mode to be used. All members should be encouraged to have their say, even if only to agree with someone else. People who are not talking may hold a much different opinion than those who are making their views known. If a decision is made only on the basis of what is said by the most vocal people, it may be no more of a consensus than taking a vote and deciding by majority rule. As a matter of fact, it could be less so, since the dissenters have not even registered negative votes.

Even if a vote will be taken, the chairperson should not call for it until all participants have given their opinions. Quieter people should be asked to state their ideas. Once people become truly invested in consensus seeking, it is common to see many members asking for comments from one another.

BEING ENCOURAGING

Dinkmeyer and Losoncy (1980) described characteristics of encouragement. These are attributes which would tend to foster the development of consensus. They include:

- effective listening;
- focusing on positives;
- cooperating;
- accepting;
- using hope and humor;
- being both stimulated and stimulating;
- recognizing effort and improvement;
- being interested in feelings; and
- valuing others.

These characteristics may already be a part of your personality. If you want to nurture their development, find a role model to emulate. Learning these skills can best be done by focusing on one at a time. As you become comfortable in manifesting one or two of these skills, you will easily move into expressing the others.

NURTURING EFFECTIVE THINKING

In an earlier book (Schoolcraft, 1984), I described some of the skills used in nurturing effective thinking. These are also relevant to promoting consensus development.

Making expectations explicit: Describe the limits and clarify what must be accomplished.

Risking and persevering: Try and stick with it.

Expanding perceptions: Use all your senses and qualities; really look at the situation.

Challenging assumptions: Avoid unwarranted assumptions.

Suspending judgement: Reserve criticism as long as possible.

Fostering self-esteem: Increase people's good feelings about themselves and protect their self-esteem.

Being patient: Allow time for incubation of ideas.

Tolerating ambiguity: Allow for uncertainty and confusion while people think over a matter.

STRATEGIES

Some ways of building consensus include conducting surveys; having discussions outside of the meetings at which decisions will be made; promoting closeness among group members outside the meetings as well as in them; defusing negative interactions; and rewarding the group for accomplishing consensus.

Surveys of the interested faculty members will help to clarify concerns and goals outside of meetings. If these are handled informally, people will usually feel fairly comfortable in sharing their ideas. When you ask others to respond to a survey, make sure they know why you're collecting the information and what you're going to do with it.

Discussing issues outside of meetings gives people more freedom to speak their mind without the time constraints often enforced within a meeting structure. People have time to mull over their ideas and get a sense of what others think. Doing things as a group outside of meetings in a social, or at least informal, context helps to build group identity. People begin to know each other better and develop a sense of concern for one another. The better committee members understand each other, the easier it will be for them to work toward consensus in a group. They will be more willing to listen and consider the opinions of their colleagues.

When committee members get into negative interchanges, the chairperson or fellow members need to help diffuse the negativity. This doesn't mean that an intervention is necessary when people may get angry or engage in heated debate. I don't consider that negative. It *becomes* negative when people are not listening to one another or when they are overtly or covertly demeaning each other. This behavior must be stopped as quickly as possible, preferably by a redirection of the discussion. If such interactions persist, relationships can be permanently damaged.

The group should be rewarded for reaching consensus. This reward can be as simple as praising the group when consensus occurs, or by more substantial actions when an issue has been of major concern. For example, a special activity, or some other supportive gesture on the part of the chairperson or the dean, will help to reinforce the value of the faculty members working together in a constructive manner.

TAKING MINUTES

The purpose of taking minutes is to document that the meeting was held and to record the actions taken by the group. Generally, it is not appropriate to record the discussion that occurred. All that needs to be recorded are the actions taken and decisions made (Robert, 1967).

Personal opinions should not be recorded. Either full names or the last name and first initial should be used to designate individuals. Titles such as "Mr.," "Ms.," or "Dr." are usually not used. It is helpful to prepare minutes so that it is easy to identify specific matters of business. This can be done by using headings as well as underlining or bold type. Table 8.2 shows a list of the components of minutes. Table 8.3 shows a sample of minutes from the meeting

Table 8.2

Components of Minutes

Name of the organization
Name of the committee
Date and time of meeting
Place of meeting
Names of members present, with indication of who was chairing
Names of members absent (usually the reason is not recorded)
Minutes of the last meeting
    Indicate if they were read and approved
    Include any corrections
All motions (except for any which were withdrawn)
    Name of the maker of each motion
    Outcome, i.e., whether the motion was passed or defeated
Summarized reports (unless written reports are appended)
Appointments of subcommittees
Time of adjournment
Signature of secretary or recorder

Vixman (1967, p. 166)

which might have resulted from the sample agenda in Table 8.1 (see p. 106). There may be a specific format required by your institution, in which case you should comply with that.

CONCLUSION

Committees form the backbone of a school and university, they get the work done which makes teaching and learning possible. If you intend to remain in academia, you should serve on a variety of committees over time. This will not only give you a broad perspective of the way academia works, but will increase your value to the institution.

Table 8.3

Minutes

ALPHA BETA SCHOOL OF NURSING
FACULTY AFFAIRS COMMITTEE
AGENDA

DATE AND TIME   February 11, 1993, 10:00 AM

PLACE   Conference Room, 3rd floor

PRESENT   David Duncan   Moira Pauley
                Linda Goldstein   Maria Rodriguez
                Angela Miller, Chair Sharon Taylor

ABSENT   Karen Montgomery

CALL TO ORDER   The meeting was called to order by Angela Miller, Chair.

MINUTES   The minutes of January 14, 1993, were approved with the following correction. On page 2, under Old Business, Search Committee, there were *three* C.V.s submitted, not *two*.

OLD BUSINESS   *Agency Workshop*: David Duncan reported on the plans for the workshop. The announcement has been developed and is being printed. The dean agreed to do one of the break-out sessions on conflict resolution. All of the other speakers were already set. Lunch will be catered by Bartley's Buffets. D. Duncan will ask for volunteers from the faculty to work at the registration table. Karen Montgomery will be in charge of that.
                Search Subcommittee: Sharon Taylor presented a written report (attached). She reminded all committee members that the first interview will be on February 20. She will circulate the schedule for the day as soon as the dean approves it.
                Updates for Faculty Handbook: The updates for the handbook were discussed. David Duncan moved that we accept the updates on faculty committee responsibilities and the copyright rules. The updates were accepted

Continued on next page

Table 8.3   (Continued)

	by consensus. Linda Goldstein pointed out that the policy on faculty and student handling of potentially hazardous patient body fluids needs to be updated in relation to current CDC guidelines. She agreed to review the policy and submit a revision for consideration at the next meeting.
NEW BUSINESS	*Position Descriptions*: Angela Miller informed the committee that the dean wants us to review the position descriptions for the coordinators of the professional practice lab and media resources. Linda Goldstein and Maria Rodriguez volunteered to work on this. They will ask Sue Jones and Doreen Goodall, the current coordinators, for input. They will try to have these done by the April meeting.
	Social Affairs: Moira Pauley, chair of the sub-committee, reported on the survey about what sort of event the faculty want for the end of the year celebration. Most of the faculty liked the catered luncheon we had at Christmas and would like to do the same in May. Several suggested a pool party at the Faculty Club. M. Rodriguez moved we have a pool party at the Faculty Club with a catered meal. The motion was accepted by consensus.
	Secretaries Day: We discussed appropriate gifts to give the secretaries in April. M. Rodriguez moved that we spend $15 on each one. The motion passed. M. Rodriguez and S. Taylor volunteered to get the gifts.
NEXT MEETING	A. Miller reminded the committee that the next regular meeting will be on March 11, 1993. The Search Subcommittee will meet on February 20 after the candidate leaves.
ADJOURNMENT	The meeting was adjourned at 11:25 AM.
RECORDED BY	*Moira Pauley* Moira Pauley

REFERENCES

Dinkmeyer, D., & Losoncy, L. E. (1980). *The encouragement book.* Englewood Cliffs, NJ: Prentice-Hall.

Robert, H. M. (1967). *Rules of order.* New York: Jove.

Schoolcraft, V. (1984). Effective and creative thinking. In (Ed.) V. Schoolcraft, *Nursing in the community* (pp. 147-166). New York: Wiley.

Vixman, R. (1967). Guide and commentary to *Rules of order,* by H. M. Robert. New York: Jove.

NINE

Documenting Accomplishments and Preparing for Advancement

•••••••••••••••••••••••••••••••••

Academia is one place where you can't stand still, even if you want to stay in the same place. In order to keep most faculty positions, you must demonstrate a consistent pattern of growth and development as a professional person. In order to progress in rank, you must meet increasingly demanding criteria. To gain tenure or a continuing contract, you must meet standards expected of a faculty member to whom the university will make such long-term commitments. It will always be your responsibility to know the relevant criteria for advancement and to be able to demonstrate that you have met these standards.

Although tenure is a common feature of academic institutions, some universities use other methods. Tenure and these other structures provide for a probationary period for faculty as well as for later security. Some schools have a system of contracts with gradually increasing lengths. The latter will be described in more

117

detail below; the term "tenure" will be used to connote this process even if that is not the name used within some systems.

PURPOSES

The purposes of this chapter are to help you to:

- identify requirements for faculty ranks;
- maintain appropriate documentation to be considered for advanced ranks, tenure, and similar long-term institutional commitments; and
- maintain a current curriculum vitae.

ACADEMIC RANKS

Your level of education, teaching experience, and other relevant personal attributes will help to determine your rank when you are offered a teaching position. The specific criteria vary from one university to another. Research-oriented universities with strong national reputations will differ from those in small liberal arts colleges. If you held an advanced rank at one of the latter institutions, you might be offered a lower rank if you moved to one of the larger or more prestigious universities.

Even before you accept a position, you might want to review the institution's criteria for promotion and tenure. This will help you to be aware of what you will be expected to accomplish in order to achieve your goals within that institution. If the criteria are more rigorous than you choose to accept, your term on the faculty could not last beyond a certain point. However, that may meet your goals. For example, you might accept a position as a junior faculty member in a highly competitive university simply for the experience.

Academic rank is the means by which accomplishments in the areas of teaching, research, and service are recognized and rewarded. The usual expectation is that once a person achieves a certain rank, that person will continue to develop professionally in order to become eligible for the succeeding ranks.

Initial Appointment

There are some general expectations for the initial appointment which are fairly common within all institutions.

Academic Degrees

In most universities, even the rank of Assistant Professor requires a doctoral degree. However, in some institutions, nursing faculty may have attained this rank without the doctorate. As doctorally prepared faculty in nursing become more available, more stringent criteria will be applied to our discipline.

Teaching Experience

Associate Professors or Professors are usually expected to have teaching experience. This could vary from about three years for Associate Professor to nine or ten for Professor.

Achievements

To be appointed at one of the higher ranks, a faculty member will be expected to have been recognized in his or her field. For Associate Professor, this might include regional activities and some publications. For Professor, this might include national or international recognition and demonstration of leadership within the discipline.

PROMOTION

Your institution will have published criteria for advancement. You should look these over, if you have not already done so, and consider what you need to do in order to advance to the next rank. This will not only help you to perform at your best, but it will also guide you in accumulating the documentation you will need to support such an advance. Some of the typical criteria considered for achievement are given here. The main reason I am including these is so that you can appreciate the similarity among universities. Obviously, you will need to consider those of your own institution to guide you in a more specific fashion.

Teaching Effectiveness

Even in research-oriented universities, there will probably be some expectation that a faculty member teach and that this will be done effectively. This will be evaluated in a variety of ways including self-student, and peer evaluation.

Scholarly and/or Creative Achievement

University faculty members are expected to contribute to the advancement of knowledge within their disciplines through research and scholarly writing. These contributions are expected to be recognized as such by the individual's discipline.

Professional and Public Service

Faculty members are expected to contribute to their professional societies through membership and leadership. They are expected to make contributions to the community by serving in roles related to their professional expertise as well as volunteering in other capacities.

University Service

Faculty members are expected to contribute to the university and the school of which they are a part by serving on committees and participating in ways that sustain and enhance the value of university life.

Professional Development

Faculty members are expected to continue to develop their own knowledge and skills through participation in professional meetings, symposia, and similar activities. If continuing education is mandated within the state where nursing faculty practice, they are expected to demonstrate compliance with the legal requirements for such activities.

TENURE AND LONG-TERM CONTRACTS

Tenure is a fairly common feature of universities. The original principle of tenure was to protect faculty so that they could pursue truth without fear of losing their position. For example, faculty members with tenure are free to speak publicly about their political beliefs and can not be relieved of their positions even if their opinions differ from those of the university administration. Another protection is that faculty members may teach what they think should be taught in their courses; they are free to speak the truth as they see it. This is the essence of academic freedom.

As universities and society have evolved, the standard of academic freedom has been applied to protect all faculty, not only those with tenure. However, tenure has survived because guaranteed jobs are one way of attracting and holding faculty. In reality, some professors have lost their jobs because their institutions simply could no longer sustain all the faculty members who had tenure, due to financial problems or to the substantial dwindling of students within certain fields.

It is beyond the scope of this chapter to offer the pros and cons of the tenure system. I will briefly state that some people feel the system has outlived its original purpose. They believe it entitles some faculty members to stop working as hard to meet standards, because they are assured a position no matter what they do.

Tenure can also alter people's behavior. People who plan to apply for tenure may compromise their values and refuse to take stands, either to win the support of those who may make tenure decisions or to avoid drawing negative attention to themselves. Furthermore, once people have tenure, they may not investigate other opportunities which would allow for growth, because they fear giving up the security.

When I left my last position to accept my present one, I gave up tenure to come into a system without it. When I told the faculty that, they were stunned. They reacted as if I were taking a chance on never being secure again in a job. I said, "Welcome to the real world!"

Another university system is one in which faculty members have one or more probationary contracts while they and the university get to know each other. After a certain time, the faculty member may apply for a continuing contract. This process requires that the faculty member meet criteria similar to those for tenure. However, the institution and the individual are making shorter-term commitments to one another. In reality, after the initial continuing contract, reviews of the faculty members may become somewhat perfunctory; but if there is a serious problem with a person, the university is in a better position to deal with it than under the tenure system, which makes it much more difficult to release a faculty member, regardless of performance.

CRITERIA FOR TENURE

The criteria for tenure and continuing or long-term contracts are similar to one another. Both are organized around categories similar to those for academic rank. However, the tenure system places even more emphasis on sustained high performance and leadership in consideration of long-term employment commitments. Some universities expect faculty members to meet their specified criterion of excellence in each area. Others may call for excellence in only one or two, but accept some other level of achievement in the other criteria. The three broad areas are discussed below.

Teaching

For tenure, faculty members are usually expected to excel as teachers. They must earn outstanding evaluations from others as to their teaching expertise, and must demonstrate creativity and versatility in their teaching responsibilities. They must not only use effective teaching skills within the classroom, clinical, and other arenas, but they must also show a high degree of skill in developing teaching materials, testing techniques, and evaluation methods.

Research

Faculty members must demonstrate a consistent contribution to the advancement of knowledge in their discipline. They must have a record of completed studies, publications in refereed journals, and presentations at professional meetings. In some instances, they may be expected to receive intramural and extramural funding for their research.

Service

To be awarded tenure, faculty members are expected to have made significant contributions to professional and public service. They may be expected to have served at the minimum as committee chairs of important committees, and may be expected to serve in elected offices as well. They will need to have demonstrated involvement with their community.

DOCUMENTATION

It's easy for me to suggest what you can do to document your accomplishments. However, it is also easy for us to forget to actually do these simple things. Then when we need this information, we're at a loss to find or recreate it. Whether you just started teaching or have been doing so for a while, you may find these ideas helpful. If you already have a system that seems to be working for you, that's great. Maybe these suggestions will enhance it.

The first consideration is the system you want to use. This can be as simple as throwing everything you think might be relevant into one file folder, or as complex as a series of folders for specific categories, such as "teaching," "professional service," "community service," and so forth. When you are new to academia, you may have few things to save, so one folder will do nicely. As you extend your career, you will become more active and you may want to start breaking up your documentation into more categories. However simple or complex you decide to make your system, the key is to *use it*.

DOCUMENTS TO BE SAVED

There are many types of documents which you should save in your files. I have tried to list everything I could think of; you will probably think of others. I have organized them under the broad categories often related to promotion and tenure. You may want to put some items under several categories when they could relate to more than one. This way, you can be sure that whatever it is, it will be there when you need it.

Documents Related to Teaching

- Student evaluations of instructor and of course;
- Self-evaluations;
- Peer evaluations;
- Course syllabi you have developed;
- Exams and other evaluation tools; and
- Course materials you have developed.

Documents Related to Scholarly Achievement

- Journal articles;
- Chapters contributed to books;
- Publication information for books you wrote;
- Papers presented at professional meetings;
- Programs or meeting notices listing your presentations;
- Photographs and contents of poster presentations;
- Proposals for studies in progress;
- Letters notifying you of research grants awarded;
- Reviews of books you wrote; and
- Publications citing awards received by your books or for your research.

Professional and Public Service

- Letters appointing you to committees;
- Letters or articles citing your election to offices;
- Letters thanking you for professional service;
- Published materials developed by you in conjunction with a committee or other professional group;
- Letters appointing you for community service activities;
- Letters thanking you for community service;
- Materials developed by you as a part of community service; and
- Newspaper articles and pictures citing your service.

Professional Development

- Published programs from meetings you attended;
- Certificates for continuing education contact hours; and
- Reports of your attendance at professional meetings and what you gained from them.

Awards

- Certificates of award for achievement;
- Certificates for membership in honor societies;
- Letters notifying you of awards; and
- Photographs or photocopies of plaques or similar awards.

University and School Service

- Notices of appointments to committees;
- Letters thanking you for service;
- Articles mentioning your contributions; and
- Documents or reports you helped to produce as part of your service to the school or university.

While you are accumulating this documentation, understand that it is better to hang on to things you may never use than to discard something without a thought. For example, when you are considered for advances in rank or for tenure, committees do not generally expect you to provide solicited or unsolicited testimonials from students. However, if you get such notes or letters from students, save them with the other documents. They may prove useful, and, if not, they will warm your heart when you run across them again.

On the other hand, when you are being considered for advances in rank or for tenure, you will probably be expected to submit letters of support from colleagues both inside and outside of the university. When you request these letters from your colleagues, make sure they understand their purpose. There is nothing wrong with asking them to address specific things in their letters of support. Make sure your colleagues have a copy of your curriculum vitae and your university's criteria for the position or for tenure. A sample letter of this type is shown in Table 9.1.

KEEPING YOUR C.V. CURRENT

Another elusive task is keeping one's C.V. up to date. It's easy enough to put off adding things until something comes up for which an updated copy is needed. Increasing accessibility to word processors has probably solved this problem to some extent. However, as with saving documentation, you have still got to remember to add things in a timely manner.

If you don't maintain your own C.V., you can refer to the items of documentation described above to update it. Another method is to keep a list of events, publications, meetings, and so on. On a regular basis, once or twice a year, have this information integrated into your C.V.

Table 9.1

Letter Soliciting a Letter of Support

Alan Strickland, Ph.D.
Professor
College of Arts and Sciences
Walker University

Dear Dr. Strickland:

I am applying for an advance in rank to full professor. I would appreciate a letter of support from you. Since we taught a class together and have worked on several committees together, I think you are in a good position to speak in my behalf.

I would appreciate it if you would share your impressions of me as a teacher. Please address my skills in lecture and in seminar facilitation. You might also want to include some comments about my expertise in test development.

Please describe my work on the Faculty Affairs and the Grant and Leaves Committees. You were chair of each of those committees when I was a member. During my time on the former, we put together a new faculty handbook, for which I did the final editing work. I also helped you to do a literature review which the Grant and Leaves committee used when the leaves criteria were revised.

If you can think of other things to cite, I will appreciate your doing so. I am enclosing a copy of my current C.V. and the criteria for the rank. If I can furnish you with anything else, please let me know.

I appreciate your willingness to help me in this way. Thank you for your time and effort.

Sincerely,

Mary Lowe, R.N., Ph.D.
Associate Professor

If you have access to a word processor, keep a copy of your c.v. on the hard disk or a floppy disk that you keep handy. When you return from a meeting or see an article in print, add the appropriate information to your C.V. immediately. The copy I keep on my disk resembles the example shown in the Appendix (p. 199). If I need to print it out, either my secretary or I can input additional headings or modify the C.V. for a particular purpose.

Each time you have your C.V. printed, check it for accuracy. You can miss errors from previous printings, or unintentionally add or delete information. Be sure it's as correct and up-to-date as possible each time you use it. Put the date of your last revision somewhere in the document, such as at the end. That way, you and others can tell how complete it is.

CONCLUSION

As you proceed with a career in academia, you should maintain good records of your accomplishments through an up-to-date curriculum vitae and documents that support it. You should be aware of the criteria by which you will be considered for advances in rank and for long-term retention. This knowledge will help you to make plans and decisions for your career. At times when it is appropriate for you to apply for advances in rank or for tenure, you will be comfortable in knowing you have made wise career choices.

·············· TEN ··············

Working on a Self-Study for School Accreditation

Every school of nursing must engage in a self-study on a regular basis. There are two specific reasons that a school does this. The first is to earn or maintain approval to offer the nursing program in your state. For this purpose your faculty must periodically complete a self-study and be visited by an evaluator, who reports to the board for regulation of nursing programs in your state. The second self-study relates to initial and continuing accreditation by the National League for Nursing. In addition to these two regular activities, faculty members may be involved to some degree in completing a self-study for accreditation of the university.

PURPOSES

This chapter will help you to:

- understand the purposes of self-studies;
- collect and document information for self-studies; and
- participate appropriately during a site visit.

129

RATIONALE FOR SELF-STUDIES

STATE APPROVAL

Licensure of nurses and approval of schools of nursing are mechanisms to protect the public. The process of licensure is not designed to give the nurse the right to work, but to ensure that nurses meet the minimal requirements to be safe beginning practitioners. In the same vein, approval of nursing programs assures the public that a given school offers the preparation necessary to enable its graduates to practice safely. Each state makes its own laws governing both licensure and approval of programs. Each state board adopts its own rules, policies, and procedures for implementing these laws.

State Rules

The state board looks for a variety of things, including the following:

- educational objectives harmonious with the curriculum;
- program objectives identifying the expected competencies of graduates;
- course objectives stating expected behaviors and relating directly to the curriculum and program objectives;
- a qualified dean/director;
- licensed and appropriately prepared nursing faculty;
- adequate financial and administrative support of the nursing program by the parent institution;
- clinical experience in appropriate quantity with effective supervision by faculty;
- adequacy and appropriateness of clinical sites; and
- a minimal performance of graduates on the licensing exam.

Reports

There are two types of reports required once a school has received initial approval. The first is an *annual report*. Each state board directs the schools as to what content is expected. These reports usually include current data on numbers of students and graduates; graduates' performance on the licensing exam; faculty credentials and accomplishments; and evaluations of some programs or options within the school. This report is usually completed by the dean and/or the director of the undergraduate program.

A *self-study* followed by an evaluator's *survey visit* occurs on a regular basis, as designated by the licensing board. Each state determines the frequency of these studies, which usually occur every three or four years.

The report for the state approval agency is often prepared by the dean and other administrators in the school; the faculty are not usually as involved in this process as they are in NLN accreditation, and the report is much less extensive. The self study is a small document of around 100 pages, made up largely of tables and samples of relevant material, such as portions of course syllabi.

Survey Visits

After the study is completed, an evaluator visits the school to verify the information provided in the report. The evaluator meets with the dean or director, reviews records, examines course materials, and usually visits at least one clinical agency. Faculty usually have minimal involvement in the visit unless the dean deems it appropriate to include them or if it is a state requirement. The evaluator's role is to verify that the school is meeting the necessary criteria to maintain the state's approval to offer the program. After the visit, the evaluator submits a report along with the school's self-study. The board of nursing then makes the decision about continuing approval.

NATIONAL LEAGUE FOR NURSING

The fundamental purpose of the criteria for the evaluation of baccalaureate and higher degree programs is stated by the National League for Nursing (1989). The criteria are meant to assist programs by serving as a guide to faculty in developing and improving educational programs and as a framework for self-evaluation. Recently, Moccia (1990) discussed her views on the process of accreditation, which she sees as a way of addressing our agendas as nursing educators. One contemporary change is the move toward evaluating in terms of outcomes rather than processes. Moccia addresses the evolution and use of the criteria as opportunities to move with the times, rather than as means to control nursing curricula.

Strutz and Gilje (1990) addressed the process and give some useful guidelines for preparing for an NLN Self-Study. These authors argue that one should organize the curriculum and record keeping around the criteria, in order to reduce the stress and time consumption inherent in other approaches.

I see a subtle difference in the two approaches described above. Moccia's is a proactive approach to affecting the development and change in criteria. Strutz and Gilje describe a reactive response. These are not in conflict with one another, and certainly the two processes may coexist. I suggest that although it is helpful to be organized for an evaluation based on the current criteria, the criteria must continue to evolve in response to the development of nursing and other relevant societal concerns. However, the practical aspect of that conjunction is that we must use the given criteria at a given time to evaluate our curricula. At the time of this writing, the 1989 criteria are still widely used; but by the time this book has been published, the newer criteria will be established. My comments are based on real life experience with the earlier and similar criteria, and less with the newer criteria.

Preparing the Self-study

The preparation of the self-study report usually begins up to two years before the visit is actually scheduled. Depending on the resources available within your institution, the preparation can be organized in a variety of ways. In some large schools, one person may be appointed as the coordinator of the study and assisted by a steering committee appointed by the dean. The steering committee would establish a timetable to follow. A sample timetable is shown in Table 10.1.

The committee also allocates the assignments; and each member might become a chairperson of a task force. Each task force is assigned specific roles or focuses on specific criteria.

Task forces meet regularly to determine the data to be gathered and the means necessary to collect it. As they collect data, they begin to write the report. The coordinator and task force chairs have a lot of responsibility for the preparation of the final report, with help from the faculty.

Table 10.1

Time Table for Self-Study

FALL 1992

September	Discuss plan of approach with faculty
	Form task forces
	Set time table
October	Task forces start meeting
	Total faculty meeting
November–	
December	Task forces collect data and begin writing

SPRING 1993

January	Task forces prepare first drafts of sections
February	First draft of self-study compiled and read by all
March	Feedback to task forces
	Corrections and preparation of second draft
April	Second draft assembled and read by all
May	Corrections to dean

SUMMER 1993

| | Dean and editing task force work on final draft |

FALL 1993

September	Final draft to faculty
October	Corrections to editing task force
	Current data put into study where needed
November	Self-study read by editor
	Corrections made
	Final copy to printer
December	Self-study and supporting material mailed to NLN

SPRING 1994

January	Begin to assemble exhibit materials
March	(After contact is made with names of visitors)
	Outline a tentative schedule for visit
	Make hotel arrangements for visitors
	Send final report to NLN
April	Arrange for local transportation for visitors
	Set up exhibit room
	Arrange for typewriter and/or computer

In a smaller school, all faculty may need to be involved in order to accomplish what needs to be done. Either discrete task forces are formed, or standing committees are given criteria to work on related to their committee charges.

As the study proceeds, efforts are made to have as many people read the drafts at various stages as possible. For example, the task force working on criteria relating to the curriculum might not include people who teach a particular group of students. The task force may thus find it difficult to describe accurately how the curriculum is implemented with different students. It will be imperative that each faculty member read the study more than once to verify data pertaining to their specific responsibilities.

As the task forces are working, they should be noting what documents they will need to be used as exhibits when the visitors come to the campus. The NLN furnishes a detailed outline of the criteria with suggestions for specific materials required for this purpose. Some of the things which might be available for exhibit are listed in Table 10.2.

In addition to the task forces focusing on sets of criteria, a group should be responsible for the details of typing, reproducing, binding, and editing the document. Another group arranges for lodging and transportation of the visitors when they are on site.

The final document usually is due to NLN four months before the visit. NLN will inform your dean of the correct number of copies to be sent. Usually enough are printed that each faculty member has a personal copy.

The Site Visit

Preparing for the Visit

About a month or so before the site visit, it is helpful for the coordinator, dean, or task force to work with the faculty to prepare them for what to expect. Prior to meeting together, every faculty member should read the final report. They should bring their questions or concerns to the meeting, particularly if they are worried about weaknesses.

Regular faculty may conduct this meeting, or someone who has been a site visitor in the past may be asked to participate. This

Table 10.2

Exhibit Materials

University catalog

School bulletin

Current semester schedule of classes

Enrollment lists

Bylaws for university and school faculty

Complete faculty vitae

Notebooks containing minutes of faculty, committee, and council meetings

University and school faculty handbooks

Copies of faculty publications

Surveys and other materials used in evaluating the programs

Samples of student papers

Complete course syllabi with related course materials and exams

Agreements with clinical agencies

School budgets

Reports of NCLEX-RN results

Other items specified by the visitors

person will read the study in advance and come prepared to discuss it. She or he may raise questions typical of site visitors which may have been overlooked or ignored. This will help faculty to formulate responses which fairly reflect the nature of the school.

Carlson and Colvin (1992) describe a novel approach to this preparation session. They designed a game format to use with their faculty that stimulated interest and helped to diminish any threat involved in the site visit by framing it in a recreational setting. The participants found this a fun and effective way to learn about the process and to become familiar with what to expect from the visitors.

A videotape presentation is available from the NLN which can be used to educate both faculty and students about the process. If possible, this should be shown to every group of students, especially those who might volunteer to talk with the visitors.

Visit Schedule

The dean or the coordinator for the self-study will be asked to prepare an agenda for the site visit. This will be sent to the lead visitor who will probably make some changes to indicate how she or he prefers to proceed. As soon as the schedule is relatively firm, a copy will probably be circulated to all faculty members. A sample schedule is in Table 10.3.

The schedule for the visit includes meetings with university and school administrators, observations of teaching, review of records and exhibits, and meetings with students, alumni, and faculty. One person or several may be responsible for arranging for people to meet with the visitors as scheduled. The very least you can expect is to be there when faculty meet with the visitors, so this date and time should be on your calendar. It is also possible that a site visitor may come to observe your teaching.

The Visitors

Accreditation visitors have been selected from volunteers who have been in academia for several years. To qualify, they have to have taught and be currently involved in a school of nursing. They attend an instructional session to learn their responsibilities and the manner in which visits are conducted. The lead visitor is someone who has participated as a member of a visiting team several times.

Prior to the appointment of the visitors, your dean will receive a list of all the possible candidates. The visitors for your school will not be people from your own state, but they will be faculty at schools similar to yours in terms of size, affiliation, and region. Since their service is voluntary, their expenses are paid, but they receive no remuneration.

The role of the visitors is to act as our colleagues in helping us to evaluate our programs. They are not there to try to catch you in a mistake or to find something negative. You can look at them as consultants; they will review your written study and investigate

Table 10.3

Schedule for Site Visit

TUESDAY

8:30 AM – 9:30 AM	Dean
10:00 AM – 11:00 AM	President
11:00 AM – 12:00 N	Vice President for Academic Affairs
12:00 N – 1:00 PM	Lunch with dean and associate deans
1:00 PM – 2:00 PM	Registrar
	Librarian
	Admissions
2:00 PM – 3:00 PM	Associate dean, undergraduate
	Associate dean, graduate
3:00 PM – 4:00 PM	Groups of students:
	Generic undergraduate students
	Career mobility students
	Graduate students
4:00 PM – 7:00 PM	Graduate classes

WEDNESDAY

9:00 AM – 12:00 N	Lecture classes, undergraduate
7:00 AM – 3:30 PM	Clinical classes, undergraduate
1:00 PM – 3:00 PM	Practice laboratory, undergraduate

THURSDAY

9:00 AM – 10:00 AM	Vice President for Business Affairs
	Vice President for Student Affairs
10:00 AM – 12:00 N	Total nursing faculty

FRIDAY

10:00 AM	Report from NLN visiting team to:
	Dean and faculty, School of Nursing
	University administration

the evidence on-site to support what you have written. They will make assessments of your strengths and weaknesses, and will recommend to the NLN review board what action should be taken in terms of accreditation.

The visiting team is made up of people who have a background in the programs in your school. If you have only an undergraduate program on one campus, you will probably have two visitors, both of whom teach in or administrate undergraduate programs of their own. If you have a graduate program, a third visitor, who is part of a graduate program, will participate. If you have satellite campuses or other off-campus offerings, a fourth visitor may be assigned to help evaluate those things.

I've been through three NLN self-studies and site visits, becoming more involved with each one as I gained seniority and responsibility in my respective institutions. The most recent one culminated in a site visit in 1992. At that time, we had four visitors: an excellent group of colleagues, who were gracious to work with. They were extremely helpful to us, and I was astonished at how hard they had to work.

The Visit

Before the visitors arrive, it's a good idea to read the self-study one more time to be aware of everything it contains. The visitors might ask you about something in the self-study, although they will usually stick to the things for which you're primarily responsible.

After all the preparation of the self-study, the visit itself seems to go by in the wink of an eye. While the visitors are on campus, you may be relatively unaware of them, unless they visit your class or your clinical site. When you have the opportunity to talk with them, you should remember that they are your colleagues, and not your judges. Try to relax, answer their questions, provide them with opportunities to talk to students and staff, and be cordial.

The visitors usually meet with the faculty as a group twice, first to ask questions and then to discuss the study. If they have questions about the rationale behind the study, they will expect any of the faculty members to be able to explain it. If there are things they think are weaknesses or problems, they will give the faculty an opportunity to discuss these concerns. If faculty have already identified the same problems, you can tell the visitors what is being done to solve them.

At the end of the visit, the visitors meet again with the faculty, as well as with the dean and other university administrators. At this meeting, they will read their report and state their recommendations. They will state the ways in which they think you have not met the criteria, as well as those ways in which you have. They will state what their recommendation will be to the board concerning accreditation or reaccreditation.

Currently, visitors are expected to make recommendations concerning accreditation. In the past, they have been responsible only for verifying the information contained in the self-study. Their report and recommendations are submitted with copies of the self-study to the review board at NLN. This board consists of other nursing educators who are within the same types of educational programs as yours. They make the final determination of the accreditation status of the school.

CONCLUSION

One criterion of a profession is that it is responsible for the oversight of its own programs for producing practitioners within its discipline. Self-studies are meant to be growth-producing activities. They give faulty the opportunity to examine what they are doing and to identify areas of concern. Although at times the process seems onerous, it is an opportunity to be responsible for ourselves and what we offer our students.

REFERENCES

Carlson, D. S., & Colvin, M. K. (1992). Making a challenge out of an NLN visit: Any more questions? *Nurse Educator, 17*(4), 27–29.

Moccia, P. (1990). Accreditation: Quality for all to see. *Nursing & Health Care, 11*, 362, 364.

National League for Nursing (1989). *Guidelines for preparation of the self-study report* (Pub. No. 15–1955). New York: National League for Nursing.

Strutz, R., & Gilje, F. (1990). How to prepare for an NLN self study. *Nursing & Health Care, 11*, 363, 365–366.

ELEVEN

Writing Effectively

Writing is an important skill in academia. You must be able to express yourself well in memoranda, reports, and manuscripts for publication. As with any skill, writing improves with practice. Some people feel they write well enough and make no effort to improve their abilities. Others, feeling they do not write well, try to avoid the activity rather than to try to develop their skills. Even experienced writers improve their ability every time they write, especially if their work is critiqued.

When I started writing for publication, I already had a fairly good style. However, my experience with both my previous books has shown me that there is always room for improvement. Although I would not have anticipated it, I actually enjoyed the opportunity to have my work edited by professionals. Each time, this has been a positive experience. It can be somewhat threatening to submit your work to this kind of perusal, but if you are willing to give the process a chance, you will find it is a gratifying opportunity.

PURPOSE

The purpose of this chapter is to help you to identify and improve the skills you need to write effectively.

WRITING SKILLS

The following suggestions are repeated from my earlier book (Schoolcraft, 1989). They are guidelines I have developed over the years as I have read about writing and have practiced writing myself.

1. Make and Follow an Outline

This is one of the most basic techniques taught in English classes, yet it seems to be ignored by most people once they actually start writing anything outside of school. An outline helps you to organize your thoughts. It gives you a sense of what should be included and in what order each topic should be addressed.

2. Use Simple Declarative Sentences

Your thoughts will be conveyed more effectively if you state them as directly as possible. Complex sentences with many clauses can become confusing and difficult to follow.

3. When In Doubt About How Something Sounds, Throw It Out

If something sounds too pompous or confusing, it probably is.

4. Avoid Pretentious Touches, such as Literary Quotations, That Don't Advance the Reader's Understanding of Your Subject

5. Avoid Slang and Other Colloquialisms

This detracts from your message, and what you have written will seem out of date within a few years.

6. When You've Made Your Point, Stop

7. A Cumbersome, Ambiguous, or Confusing Sentence Can Usually Be Improved

There are three ways to approach this problem. Break the sentence up into more than one sentence; shorten it, rather than add to it; or drop the sentence altogether.

8. Use the Same Tense Throughout Unless There's a Particular Reason to Do Otherwise

9. Use the Active Voice

Unless the recipient of the action is more important than the person or thing doing the acting, select the active voice. For example, "The charge nurse on the evening shift instructed all patients on the preoperative regimen" is clearer than "The patients were instructed on the preoperative regimen." In this case, the person who did the instructing is important.

There are some situations in which the apparent object is more important than the apparent subject. The passive case is appropriate in these cases. For example, "Every patient was nauseated by this protocol for chemotherapy" is more effective than "This protocol for chemotherapy nauseated every patient."

10. Make Sure the Subject and Verb of Each Sentence Agree in Number

One way to check for this is to ignore all the words between your subject and verb, and read what's left. For example, take the sentence: "The investigators found that a group of strangers *is* more likely to share such experiences than *is* a group of friends." The subject in each clause is "group," and not "strangers" or "friends." The verb in each case should be "is," and not "are" as you might think if you don't read it carefully.

11. Avoid Sexist Language

Although you may find that avoiding sexist language is sometimes cumbersome, you must do so in order to be considerate of your readers. One way of doing this is to use plural nouns and pronouns. For example, "Each nursing student will teach her client how to take her child's temperature" is sexist unless all students and parents are always female. Another way to express it would be "All nursing students will teach their clients to take their children's temperatures."

12. Refer to Yourself in the Third Person in Formal Writing, Unless the Situation Calls for a First-person Account

I chose to use the first person in this book, because I want this to have the tone of one colleague talking to another. However, if I were describing the outcome of a research project, I would use the third person.

13. Start Writing and Putting Ideas Together Without Worrying About How it Sounds

If you try to write perfectly from the beginning, you won't accomplish much. You can hone and polish what you've written after you have down the gist of what you want.

14. After Writing Something, Leave It Alone for a Few Days

You may be surprised to find how well or how badly you have written something if you give yourself some time to reconsider it. When you review it from a fresh perspective, you may have a better sense of what you really want to say.

15. If You Feel You Need a Thesaurus to Write Something, You're Probably Trying Too Hard

Generally, straightforward, everyday language is preferable for communicating your message. The only time I resort to a thesaurus is when I'm writing something in which a precise word is needed. This usually concerns me only when I'm writing something like a resolution for other people to adopt.

16. If You're Unsure of the Spelling of a Word, or if You're Trying to Spell a Word You Don't Usually Use, Look It Up in a Dictionary

Most of us have access to word processing programs that include spell checkers. These have been a boon to all writers.

17. The More You Want to Keep a Particular Passage Because It Sounds So Wonderful to You, the More You Should Consider Dropping It

Anything that makes you feel this way probably has a lot of ego invested in it and may actually detract from your reader's appreciation of your point.

18. The Greater the Sense of Accomplishment Upon Completing the First Draft of a Work, the Greater the Need For Revision

This is particularly true for novice writers. As I have stated before, almost all initial attempts at written work can be improved.

19. If you Have Trouble Writing a First Sentence, Start Somewhere Else

Sometimes if you start in the middle, after you have completed what you want to write, the first sentence will actually be there. If not, you will better be able to decide the best way to introduce what will follow.

20. If You Have Trouble Writing a Last Sentence, You've Probably Already Written It

This is akin to #6—the notion that when you have made your point, you should stop. Trust your reader to recognize that the final point has been made.

21. Break Up Your Piece With Headings and Subheadings.

Use italics and underlining for emphasis or as attention-getters. Even in memos, this can help to convey your points more effectively. In a major piece of writing, it is essential.

22. Write Something Every Day, Even if it Isn't Directly Related to Your Major Writing Project

This helps you to keep practicing the skill of writing, and you may find that you easily move into this phase of your major project.

23. Don't Be Afraid to Let Someone Else Read and Edit Your Work

Choose someone who is a good writer and whose judgment you respect. You do not have to make all the changes such a person suggests, but you will still find other ways of better expressing yourself. The more important the thing you're writing is, the more you need to follow this step. I frequently have someone else read even my short memos and notices to make sure they answer all the questions someone would have in receiving the communication.

24. Always Proofread Your Work

Even if you use a spell checker, words may be spelled correctly, yet still be out of context. You may have inadvertently dropped words or whole sentences. You may want to ask someone else to proofread for you, so that you don't make the same errors in reading that you did in writing.

25. Get One Or Two Handbooks On English

There are many handbooks available that are more accessible than texts for helping you with questions about syntax, grammar, and usage. One of the best and easiest to use resources is the *Elements of Style* by Strunk and White (1979). A more extensive reference that is also convenient to use is Johnson's *The Handbook of Good English* (1982).

26. Choose Your Typist Carefully

For memos and other internal documents, this is not a big issue, since you will probably have access to secretaries to do typing. However, for other written work, you may hire a typist. Make sure the typist understands all the parameters that need to be followed to suit you or the criteria demanded by the recipient of your work.

27. If You Can Type, Consider Using a Word Processor

Although it takes time to become comfortable with composing while you're typing, once you become accustomed to it, it can actually facilitate your writing. You can easily rearrange content and print out a new hard copy that is easy for you to review. I started writing on a typewriter when I was in my doctoral program. I eventually got a word processor and was very pleased with how helpful it was, both for my first book and for my dissertation.

28. If a Particular Style Is Required, Get the Appropriate Manual Or Guidelines and Learn How to Use It

Most publications require a particular style. This information is usually published in the journal itself. For other major writing projects, consult the recipient's office to find out what style is appropriate.

29. If You're Using References, Make Bibliography Cards On All Articles, Books, and Personal Interactions As Soon As Possible

Write the citation in the same style you intend to use for the finished product. This saves time and frustration. Even if you think it's unlikely that you will use a particular reference, make a card. It's better to have cards you don't need than to have to hunt for the citation if you need it later.

WRITING MEMOS AND LETTERS

Your primary concern before you write a letter or a memo is whether or not the written communication is necessary. People frequently send written communication simply because they don't wish to interact with the recipient. If it is possible to talk with the other person face-to-face or by telephone, that is usually preferable. However, letters and memos may be useful when you are trying to communicate with people whom you do not see on a regular basis. Letters and memos are also helpful if you need a written record that you have communicated the content involved.

The key principle in writing effective memos and letters is to avoid distractions and tangents within them, and to keep them simple.

TONE

Bates (1985) has written an excellent book about communicating in the business world. *Writing with Precision* carries the subtitle

"How to write so that you cannot possibly be misunderstood." This is an extremely useful resource. Bates discusses the importance of the tone of your professional correspondence. Some of the important things to avoid are:

> Don't write in a way that angers or frustrates your reader.
>
> Don't insult the reader's intelligence.
>
> Don't say anything that might be construed as a putdown.
>
> Don't preach or pontificate; keep off the soapbox and out of the pulpit.
>
> Don't talk down to the reader.
>
> Don't use unsuitable humor or backslapping familiarity.
>
> Don't use sarcasm, exaggeration, or attempts at satire. ... You will almost inevitably be misunderstood or misconstrued by most of your readers.
>
> Don't make dogmatic, highly opinionated, aggressive, or smartalecky pronouncements.
>
> Don't "argue" with the reader—that is, don't blatantly accuse the reader of being wrong, of having misunderstood, or of not being clear.
>
> Don't sound off at the reader.
>
> Don't write when you are angry; or if you do, tear up your letter, don't mail it!
>
> Don't pass the buck; if you made a mistake, admit it. (pp. 80-81)

Sometimes, colleagues end up angry at one another over nothing more than a memo which neglects one or more of the points listed above. Tables 11.1 and 11.2 show examples of the same content conveyed in two different ways. After looking at the first table and before you look at the second, try rewriting the same memo in a more appropriate tone.

The memo in Table 11.1 casts blame, downgrades the recipients, and disavows any responsibility on the part of the writer for whatever happened. The second memo conveys the same information in terms of the expected performance, but the writer conveys an empathetic, friendly tone that avoids casting blame. The writer also conveys an empathetic understanding of the plight of a new faculty member and a friendly offer of further assistance.

Simplicity

You should make your point as quickly and briefly as possible while still conveying all pertinent information. Tables 11.3 and 11.4 show two examples of a memo, the first poorly written, and

Table 11.1

Memo Cast in an Inappropriate Tone

TO:	Darrell Blank, Pam Meyers, Milly Winedock
FROM:	Curtis Lawrence
RE:	Faculty Responsibilities

I know you're new to the faculty this year, but even new faculty should know their responsibilities. When I ask you for test items by a particular day, I expect you to have them in my box by 4 PM of that day. I think you were told this during the orientation. Even though you have a lot of new things to learn, I don't think this is all that complicated an expectation.

Table 11.2

Memo Cast in an Appropriate Tone

TO:	Darrell Blank, Pam Meyers, Milly Winedock
FROM:	Curtis Lawerence
RE:	Test Items

I know that being a new faculty member is complicated, and it is easy to overlook something because everything is new. I may not have made my expectations clear about the test items you are preparing for our exam. Please get them to me as soon as possible. In the future, I will give you a specific date and time for when I need them. If there is anything else I can help you with as you become oriented, please let me know.

the second of better quality. In Table 11.3, the author is slow to come to her point, which is to call a meeting. The heading does not indicate that the memo is actually a meeting notice, and a lot of the language is negative, almost damning the recipients before a discussion has even ensued. Even the final statement that "Everyone should be there" is not a clearly stated expectation as to attendance.

In Table 11.4, the heading makes clear the intent of the memo. Its purpose is stated in a simple declarative sentence. No implications are included of a lack of compliance on anyone's part, and

Table 11.3

Ineffectively written memo

TO:	Pediatric Nursing Faculty
FROM:	Mary Lowe, Coordinator
RE:	Clinical Skills

It has come to my attention through some meetings, as well as personal contacts, that there is some discrepancy between faculty members in terms of expectations for competency of clinical skills in the pediatric areas. Apparently some faculty have neglected to review the guidelines given in the syllabus for the competency levels. If there is doubt, faculty should consult the guidelines or discuss this with me.

Because of this problem, a meeting is called for. At this meeting, competencies will be discussed. It will be held in Room 210 on Thursday, October 21, 1-3 P.M. Everyone should be there.

Table 11.4

Effectively written memo

TO:	Pediatric Nursing Faculty
FROM:	Mary Lowe, Coordinator
RE:	Meeting to Discuss Clinical Competencies

I am calling a meeting on Thursday, October 21, from 1–3 P.M. to be held in Room 210. The purpose of this meeting is to discuss the clinical competencies expected of our students and to ensure that all clinical faculty have similar expectations. I expect everyone to attend. If you cannot, please notify me in advance. I look forward to seeing you then.

the author's expectation about attendance is stated directly. The final sentence conveys respect and friendliness in contrast to the judgmental flavor of the other memo.

The same considerations in writing memos should be followed in composing letters. Usually letters are much more formal, and are more likely to be used in communicating outside the institu-

Table 11.5

Poorly written letter

Ellen Prather, MSN, RN
Marvin Psychiatric Hospital
11200 N.E. 70th Street
Miami, FL 33181

Dear Ms. Prather:

In regards to our discussion by telephone on August 18, I would like to follow up with this letter to avoid any misunderstanding about what we agreed to in respect to the clinical placement for my clinical students. There will be 10 students in the group, which will include two males. These are junior students who have completed all their clinical except for psychiatric nursing, community health, and management. For most of them, this will be their first experience in a psychiatric setting. I am sure you know how crucial the attitudes of you and your staff will be in ensuring that the students have a good experience.

We will be in the clinical area on Wednesdays and Thursdays from 6:45 AM to 2:00 PM each day. I will have a postclinical conference with them from 2:00 to 3:00 on each day. You need to arrange for a conference room for my use.

Sincerely,

---

tion or for very formal situations, such as supporting someone for a promotion.

Tables 11.5 and 11.6 show examples of a common letter you might write to confirm clinical arrangements. The writer in Table 11.5 seems to imply that trouble is expected. There is also somewhat of an officious tone rather than simple delivery of factual information. This letter does not include some of the most crucial data, such as the inclusive dates, and the writer does not properly thank the recipient for her help. Include only the information required; extraneous issues such as the number of men in the group or what clinical the students have already had, are not necessary.

The content of Table 11.6 is presented in a more straightforward manner. Extraneous information is omitted. The request for help in arranging for a conference room is made in a polite tone, and the writer expresses appropriate appreciation for the assistance being given.

Table 11.6

Well-Written Letter

Ellen Prather, MSN, RN
Marvin Psychiatric Hospital
11200 N.E. 70th Street
Miami, FL 33181

Dear Ms. Prather:

This letter is to follow up on our August 18 telephone conference. My clinical group of 10 students will be on your units every Wednesday and Thursday from 6:45 AM to 2:00 PM. Their first day will be September 8 and their last day will be December 10. They will not be there either day Thanksgiving week.

Each day, I need a conference room from 2:00 to 3:00 PM. I appreciate your arranging for a room for us.

The first day will be orientation for the students. I will contact you and the charge nurses about meeting with the students and sharing what you think is important for them.

I appreciate your help in allowing me and my students to come to your facility. This has been a good experience in the past, and I am looking forward to working with all of you.

Sincerely,

LETTERS OF RECOMMENDATION

Another commonly written letter in academia is the reference for a colleague or a former student. Such letters may be requested when the person involved is being considered for a new position, a promotion, an advance in rank, tenure, an honor, or an award. Such letters should include adjectives, adverbs, and judgements.

If you write a flat, unmodified letter of recommendation, it will appear that you are not really trying to convey a positive impression of the person involved. On the other hand, it may actually be your intent not to sound supportive. If I don't feel I know someone well enough to write a genuinely positive letter, or if for any reason I do not want to write such a letter, I decline to do so.

There are some former students or colleagues whom I remember positively, although I may be unable to recall specific incidents from our association. When writing letters of recommendation, I ask them to remind me of things they feel are pertinent from when we worked together.

The following is a list of suggestions for writing a letter of recommendation.

- If there is a position description or a list of criteria related to the purpose of the letter, request copies in order to adequately respond;
- Ask the person involved if there are specific comments you should make;
- Address as directly as possible those qualities in the person which apply to the purpose of the letter;
- Make clear your role in relation to the person so that your suitability to describe them is clear;
- Give descriptive examples whenever possible;
- Use positively charged adjectives and adverbs; and
- Express specific judgments about the person's suitability for the position or honor.

Tables 11.7, 11.8, and 11.9 show letters of recommendation for a former student applying for a new position; for a former student applying for a graduate program; and for a colleague applying for tenure.

WRITING REPORTS AND POLICIES

There will be many times when you will need to write reports to account for what you are doing or to describe the outcome of a particular project. Frequently, you will be expected to produce or help to produce reports from committees. You may also be responsible for monthly and/or annual reports about your responsibilities. The general guidelines listed on pages 142–147 should give guidance in producing reports. When you write a report, you should attend to the specific content expected.

A report should be succinct and be written in language appropriate to the recipient or recipients. You should identify any data which you have used to arrive at any recommendations you have made. This data should be stated as directly and clearly as possible.

Your recommendations should be clear and connected to the data or other supporting information you have described. If ap-

Table 11.7

Reference letter for former student

Barbara Wilmont, MSN, RN
Pacific Coast Psychiatric Hospital
7000 West Parkway
Sacramento, CA 95823

Dear Ms. Wilmount:

I am writing in support of Mr. Nicholas Joseph's application for a position at your hospital. Regretfully, he and I have had limited contact for the last several years, since we moved to opposite coasts. However, I knew him well when he was my student and for a time after he graduated.

As a student, Mr. Joseph was well prepared for class and clinical experiences in psychiatric nursing. He worked well with his peers, patients, staff, and faculty. He was responsible and seemed mature beyond his years. He was active in student organizations and often took a leadership position to facilitate the work of the group. He represented the university at state and national conventions of the student nurses association. I was the faculty advisor to the group at that time and observed him to be an excellent representative and an effective participant. He was named by the faculty to *Who's Who in American Colleges and Universities*.

After he graduated, I worked with him frequently when I was supervising clinical students in psychiatric nursing. He was one of the most helpful staff members. He was effective in his clinical practice and provided an excellent role model for students to emulate. He was often available to share his experiences with students and to help them to link theory with practice. Mr. Joseph projected a caring attitude about patients which was genuine and made an impression on students.

I never heard him make a comment about another person which was disrespectful or dehumanizing. As a matter of fact, I recall one instance in which he acted as a patient and staff advocate, when one of the psychiatrists proposed a dehumanizing intervention in caring for a particular patient. Mr. Joseph appropriately asked for an explanation of the physician's plan which the physician could not provide. Subsequently, with Mr. Joseph's leadership, the staff refused to implement the tactics proposed by the physician.

Mr. Joseph's actions in the above incident were not capricious. I believe his action was as justified as if he had questioned the administration of a harmful drug. I thought his behavior was courageous. He provided a model for other nurses and for my students which I hope they never forgot. I still respect him for this action and have used it as an example in assertiveness training for nurses.

Throughout his undergraduate work, Mr. Joseph earned mostly Bs with some As. I think his record was typical of many students who are "well-rounded." He made better than average grades, and also devoted time to participating in meaningful extracurricular activities. These activities increased his leadership abilities and his breadth as a person.

I believe Mr. Joseph is well qualified for this position. I think he is a superior example of a professional person. He will do well in your institution, and I think you will be happy to have him work with you.

Sincerely,

Table 11.8

Reference Letter for Continued Education

Dear Dr. Washington:

I am writing this letter in reference to Monica Smith, who is applying for admission to your graduate program. Ms. Smith was my student in a psychiatric nursing course. I also had frequent contact with her in my role as school advisor to the nursing students' association.

Ms. Smith was an excellent student. She graduated with a 3.85 grade point average. She earned this by excelling in the classroom as well as in the clinical setting. She wrote papers that were well above the level of usual undergraduate student. Her practice in the clinical area demonstrated that she understood what she wrote and could apply it to various patients. She was conscientious in every way, and frequently went beyond minimal expectations to learn as much as she could in a setting.

I have taught graduate students and have chaired thesis committees, so I am familiar with expectations for graduate work. Ms. Smith is already writing papers at that level. She is a serious student who is interested in eventually going on for her doctorate.

Ms. Smith was secretary for the school chapter of the State Nursing Student's Association in her junior year. She served as chairperson of the state newsletter committee and as an Executive Board member for the state level in her senior year. I worked closely with her during that time. She was an effective officer and very productive as a committee chair. The group had a history of poorly produced newsletters. She was resourceful and creative in finding support and was able to produce such improved publications that the state association won a national honorable mention award.

Ms. Smith has made and will continue to make substantial contributions in her chosen field of nursing. I am proud that she is one of our graduates. You will be gratified to work with such a good student.

Sincerely,

Table 11.9

Reference Letter for a Colleague

Anthony Gonzalez, Dh.D
Chair, Rank and Promotions Committee
Walker University

Dear Dr. Gonzalez:

I am writing this letter in reference to Dr. Karen Keith, who is applying for an advance to the rank of Associate Professor. Dr. Keith has been on our faculty for three years, since she completed her doctorate. During that time, she has been primarily responsible for teaching the course "Care of the Child."

Although she had only the teaching experience which was part of her graduate program, Dr. Keith has proven to be an effective teacher. Her lectures are well organized and comprehensive. Her style in giving lectures is very good. She is able to present very complex information in a way that is accessible to all students. She varies her approach and makes good use of media to provide the students with needed content while keeping their attention.

Dr. Keith asked me to be her peer evaluator in the clinical area last year. I found her to be very effective in supervising her clinical students. She gave them extensive direction to help them to get started in the morning. She was constantly on the go, but managed to spend an appropriate amount of time with each student.

For example, she had one student who was very anxious about giving her first injection to a child. Dr. Keith talked to the student before she started the process. She was accepting of the young woman's feelings, and it was obvious that the student felt secure about being open about these feelings. Dr. Keith was gentle yet persistent in guiding the student through the steps. When they entered the child's room, Dr. Keith distracted the patient, who seemed to have no idea that the student was nervous. Dr. Keith took the lead in talking to the patient while the student started preparing for the injection. Although I could tell that Dr. Keith was watching the student carefully, she did so in such a way that she increased neither the student's nor the child's anxiety. The student was able to give the injection and, with Dr. Keith's help, quickly focused her attention on her patient. Afterwards, Dr. Keith literally patted the student on the back and congratulated her on succeeding.

I have much admiration for Dr. Keith. She is an excellent teacher who will always work to continue to be at her best in this role. She well deserves the promotion, and I am happy to encourage you to support this advance in rank for her.

Sincerely,

Table 11.10

Report

TO: Undergraduate Faculty

FROM: Student Affairs Committee

RE: Attendance Policy

The Student Affairs Committee has been charged with writing a new policy regarding classroom and clinical attendance. We reviewed the old policy and discussed the concerns of faculty teaching all the undergraduate courses.

Most of the faculty expressed more concern with clinical absences or tardiness than with attendance of lectures. That is why we are leaving the latter issue to the discretion of the course committees.

If the following policy is adopted, we recommend that it go into effect immediately. We would distribute a copy of it to every undergraduate student to replace the old policy in their student handbooks.

Policy for Attendance

Classroom attendance: The policy for classroom attendance in each course will be determined by the respective course committee. The policy will be included in the course syllabus.

Clinical attendance: Attendance is required for all clinical and laboratory sessions. Any student unable to attend or arrive on time for a clinical or laboratory session is to notify the appropriate faculty member as early as possible, no later than *one hour* before the scheduled experience. Faculty may request a physician's note to support absences reportedly due to illness.

All clinical absences and tardiness will be documented on the student's record for the course. If the student misses more than 20% of the clinical or laboratory experience, the student may be required to make up such absences. This will be at the faculty member's discretion if the faculty member thinks additional clinical experience is required for the student to satisfactorily meet the objectives of the clinical assignment.

If a student is required to make up clinical time in order to satisfy the objectives of the course, the student will pay a fee of $35 per hour for each hour of make up time required. The time must be made up prior to the published date by which grades must be submitted for the semester involved.

If absences are so excessive that time is not available for make up, the student may withdraw from the course if this is done during the withdrawal period. If the established withdrawal period has closed, the student will receive a failing grade for clinical and for the course.

If a student has been told that make up time is required, but the student believes this is unwarranted, the student should initially discuss this with the faculty member involved. If the student continues to disagree with the faculty member, she or he may appeal to the course coordinator to reconsider. If the student is still expected to make up the time and feels it is unjustified, she or he may appeal to the associate dean for the undergraduate program. The decision of the associate dean will be final.

propriate to the situation, you should also describe how the recommendations should be implemented. Table 11.10 shows an example of a report from a committee.

This sample report also demonstrates the format used for a policy statement. A policy statement should be in clear, easy-to-read English. It should specify to whom it applies, exactly what is expected, what the consequences are for noncompliance, and the recourse, if any, when the policy has not been adhered to.

Whenever I need to write a policy, I always ask someone else to read it, preferably someone to whom the policy might apply. I then ask that person to tell me what they think the policy means. I ask them who it applies to; when it is applicable; what the penalties are; and what they could do if they failed to follow the policy. This helps me to rewrite the document, if necessary.

CONCLUSION

Faculty members frequently are expected to write formal and informal documents. The skill of writing such materials is enhanced by the experience of having your work critiqued by others. With practice and intelligent assistance, you will be able to improve your ability to communicate in writing.

REFERENCES

Bates, J. D. (1985). *Writing with precision*. Washington, DC: Acropolis.

Johnson, E. D. (1982). *The handbook of good English*. New York: Facts on File.

Schoolcraft, V. (1989) *A nuts-and-bolts approach to teaching nursing*. New York: Springer.

Strunk, W., Jr., & White, E. B. (1979). *The Elements of Style*. New York: MacMillan.

TWELVE

Initiating
and Participating in
Change

Eventually you will identify things at your institution you think should be changed. In order to make appropriate changes, you need to be realistic about your abilities and about your own wisdom in wanting to make these changes. New people often bring a fresh perspective to a situation. They frequently can identify problems and suggest new solutions. What is important is their timing and wisdom in doing so.

To be frank, even though many of us may intellectually understand the above, there are few things more irritating to some of us than a new person who thinks he or she knows exactly what's wrong and how to fix it shortly after arriving. You will find that you are more likely to estrange people than to endear them to you if you aren't careful about proposing and trying to bring about changes.

PURPOSES

The purposes of this chapter are to:

- help you to identify institutional constraints and enablers in bringing about change;
- help you to identify colleagues who may facilitate or hinder your efforts; and
- help you to improve your timing and groundwork in relation to change.

CHANGE THEORY

Although change theory is a common feature of most undergraduate and graduate nursing curricula, I will review some of the concepts here to make sure we are speaking the same language.

CHANGE

Change is "any planned or unplanned alteration in the status quo in an organism, situation, or process" (Lippitt, 1973, p. 37). The classic model for change which I like to use is Lewin's (1958), which described behavior as a function of personality and environment. Therefore, changing behavior is a complicated undertaking. This helps to explain why change is so complex and often so difficult.

It is sometimes deceptively simple to sum up a complex process in a few words. Never could this be more true than when describing the process of change. Lewin's (1958) model describes three phases of change: *unfreezing*, *changing*, and *refreezing*. Lewin's words paint a useful picture. Think of a block of ice that has been frozen to resemble nothing but a huge cube. Think of that block melting over time. The time required would depend on the size of the block as well as the surrounding conditions; a huge block in a cold room would change less rapidly than a smaller block in a warm room. Add direct heat, and it would melt even faster.

Next think of the process of changing. No longer are you limited to a preformed block. Now you have a vat of fluid ready for change. While in a fluid state, you can add color and new components, such as oil, glitter, or flowers. Then you can decant the fluid into a new mold.

Refreezing starts and you may have to occasionally fine-tune your new creation. As the new shape forms, you may have to stir it to keep the new components from settling in the wrong places. Gradually, as your ice freezes, it takes on the new shape you have determined—an eagle, a swan, or a soaring spire. The time it takes to refreeze is also determined by the components, the size, and the surrounding conditions.

Unfreezing is the first step in change. The descriptive word well fits the sense of melting barriers and resistances so that the person, situation, or process can be reformed into something new. Lewin (1958) identified the effects of driving and restraining forces which affect change. Both of these concepts must be viewed objectively. There is no intrinsic value either in driving for change or for restraining change. Either one may be "best" at one time or another, but in any given situation, both must be thought of as integral parts of the process.

One of the most crucial things you must develop is an appreciation of the opposite point of view to your own when a change is proposed. Before you start arguing for your own position, you must first investigate the other. You must know it as well as your own. This will help you to advance your position, as well as to appreciate what the others think and feel in the situation. It could even change your mind about what you believe is right in the situation.

Resistance is normal when change is proposed. It is not enough for you to recognize this intellectually; you must accept the principle that it is a *normal* part of change. Resistance is not merely an inconvenience or something to be surmounted. It is a normal response by normal people. The main reason people resist change is that they feel and think that the change will have a higher cost than the benefits are worth. Their perception may be based on the interests they have in the organization as much as upon their personal interests. However, the sense of the impact of a change on personal needs and interests is usually the most significant determinant of an individual's response.

There is nothing wrong with people being motivated by self-interest. Healthy self-interest has accounted for many of the most significant advances in our society. Self-interest which leads to resistance can be very helpful in retarding growth which is too fast or not well considered. Trying to overcome resistance with brute force will usually only delay the inevitable death of an idea.

Changing is the phase in which implementation occurs. The person or organization is the most vulnerable during this phase. The planning that goes on during the unfreezing stage is crucial to helping people work through the transition from old to new. Unresolved resistance will crop up and may sabotage all the efforts made to change.

In this phase, final plans are made and efforts to change are begun. You will implement activities planned to give the people involved a sense of security and reward for participating in the change. As this work progresses, the people involved evaluate the process and may make changes in the original plans. Evaluation may result in the decision to return to the original manner of functioning or to proceed with the transition to something new.

Refreezing starts once the person or group is functioning at the desired level. You must realize that during the refreezing phase, the person or the group may return to their previous level of functioning. No matter how appropriate the proposed change seems to some in the group, the majority of the members or even the original agents of change may determine that the new proposal is less satisfactory than the old one. At any rate, refreezing occurs when the group is functioning regularly at the new level and there is no longer a sense of transition.

STRATEGIES

Zaltman and Duncan (1977) describe various change strategies in detail. They also suggest a continuum within which to fit these strategies and determine which is appropriate. The factor which determines the suitability of one approach or another is external pressure. Where there is minimal external pressure, educative strategies are useful because time is available for more gradual change effected by learning. As the external pressure comes more to bear, first facilitative and then persuasive strategies work best. When there is maximum outside pressure, power strategies must be used.

Reeducating

When time is not a factor, reeducation is the best approach. This strategy involves the "relatively unbiased presentation of fact...intended to provide a rational justification for action" (Zaltman & Duncan, 1977, p. 111). The underlying assumption is that human beings are rational and are able to change their behavior when they have the facts to support such change.

A change that has occurred gradually in schools of nursing is the adoption of a particular model from which the curriculum should emerge. This was not originally a mandate for any school, but eventually became a part of the criteria for accreditation. One way of bringing this about was to educate faculty about models and the development of curriculum based on models. To some extent, this change is still occurring as we become more sophisticated about theory and its uses.

Facilitating

According to Zaltman and Duncan (1977), facilitative strategies "make easier the implementation of changes by and/or among the target group" (p. 90). The underlying assumptions are that the group recognizes the problem; agrees that action is needed; and is open to assistance and self-help.

One example of this would be a faculty desiring to increase cultural diversity among students and faculty. These faculty members have recognized that they are influenced by their own cultural backgrounds, and realize they cannot make a change without outside assistance to identify strengths and weaknesses. Once they arrive at these conclusions, they can work well with facilitators who help to make the desired changes.

Persuading

Persuasive strategies deliberately use bias when presenting information. Although the appeal may be rational, the facts may be true or completely false (Zaltman & Duncan, 1977). This type of strategy has more obvious ethical implications than others, in the sense that deliberate efforts to mislead are a common feature.

For example, a group of people within the faculty may want a particular nursing model adopted for use as the underpinning of the curriculum. Instead of providing a well-balanced presentation of a variety of models, they deliberately present their favorite model in the best possible light. They tailor their presentation to the biases of other faculty members. When discussing other option, they leave out important information or emphasize unfavorable aspects.

Powering

Power strategies involve "the use of coercion to obtain the target's compliance. This coercion takes the form of manipulation or threat of manipulation of the target's outcomes" (Zaltman & Duncan, 1977, p. 152). To be able to use power strategies, the change agent must have the ability to control the target group's goal satisfaction. Such strategies may be used by the dean, for example, when forces outside the school dictate changes which aren't negotiable. For example, one National League for Nursing criterion for accreditation of baccalaureate programs is that all faculty must have a minimum of the MSN degree. Although faculty might be hired with only the BSN, power would be exerted to pressure those people into earning the MSN, or they would no longer remain on the faculty.

VALUES AND ETHICAL IMPLICATIONS

When you are involved in bringing about any change, you must be aware that you are determining what *should* change and *how* it should change based on your own values. Your values are not necessarily better or worse than those of the other people you want to involve in the change. Examine your values in your particular situation and consider the values of others involved. Frequently, people assume that the values of the others in a situation are misguided. To understand anyone's values, we have to know that person better.

All too often, we make conclusions about other people without first trying to understand how their value systems developed. An example of value systems in operation is given in Situation 12.1.

Situation 12.1

Clarifying Values

Tyler Lane was responsible for the RN to BSN Option in his school. He wanted to require fewer clinical courses for RNs and to replace them with standardized tests. Several other faculty members were vocal in opposing this change. Their support for their opposition was rational; they believed there was a need for the RNs to actually experience clinical practice with the different demands inherent in the baccalaureate curriculum. Tyler countered with research showing that the tests he wanted to use have in fact demonstrated a knowledge base which is comparable to that of generic BSN graduates, if not better.

Finally, Tyler decided to get to know his opponents better. Of the four most vocal, Tyler discovered that three were career ladder students themselves. They all had attended programs where they had to attend classes with generic students and had few exceptions made in their curricula. The fourth was a very young faculty member who worked the minimum amount as an RN expected of faculty. Tyler needed to understand their prejudices. Their reasons were subtler than he or anyone else might have concluded from this information.

For example, one bitter faculty member had the attitude that, "If I had to do it, so should they." The youngest of them admitted she felt uncomfortable in implying that some RNs could learn as much in practice as in an academic setting. The other two were seriously concerned about compromising the students' experience, which they felt was enriched by going through the courses rather than testing out of them.

By identifying his colleagues' biases, Tyler was in a better position to reeducate them. He helped them to look at the way in which nursing and nursing education have evolved. He acknowledged and demonstrated that he valued the sacrifices and self-doubts of his colleagues. He shared more information with them about studies supporting his approach, and got them more involved with the courses the RNs would be taking, so that the components they felt were crucial would be included.

Tyler's values were not better than those of his opponents. Theirs were as justified as his. However, when Tyler showed them respect and a willingness to understand their positions, they were much more receptive to his planned changes than if he had ignored their concerns. He gained allies in curriculum change, as well as increasing their mutual respect for the future.

IDENTIFYING A NEED FOR CHANGE

The most crucial step in making a change is to *define* what needs to be changed. Everyone involved needs to define the problem similarly and come to accept that a change is needed. Sometimes people want to make a change without being able to verify that there actually is a problem.

Often the problem is a personal one, even though the proposed change would involve more than that one person or persons concerned. The person or persons who want a change may simply want things to be different in order to feel more comfortable, but there is no real problem in terms of others in the situation. Those who want to make such changes are unlikely to meet a welcome reception. Why should others change just because you are uncomfortable? This is why many proposed changes are doomed to failure.

If you think there is a problem affecting the whole system, work with your colleagues to identify it specifically. Table 12.1 shows the process of describing a problem from a general statement of concern to a specific formulation.

Once the problem is clearly defined, the *desired outcome must be stated*. Several statements which progress from a general to a specific and measurable outcome are given in Table 12.2. Obviously, the more specific your outcome statements, the more direction you will have in accomplishing a change.

The next step is to *formulate a plan* for accomplishing the desired outcome. Depending on how complex the problem is, this plan could have many components and lengthy periods required for the stages involved. Table 12.3 gives an example of a plan which would relate to the problem and outcome statements developed in previous other tables.

INSTITUTIONAL CONSTRAINTS AND ENABLERS

Once you have developed a plan, you can begin to identify the driving forces and the resisting forces for change. In dealing with the institution, I'll call these *constraints* and *enablers*. Not surprisingly, the constraints and enablers will come from the same sources. This would include such things as:

Table 12.1

Problem Statement Formulation

The initial concern: There aren't any Blacks, Hispanics, or other minorities on the faculty.

Why this is important: The student population is ethnically diverse.

The problem statement: Students, regardless of whether they are in the majority or the minority ethnically, do not have a variety of role models on the faculty.

Table 12.2

Outcome Statements

General: There will be more faculty members from ethnic minorities.

Specific: The percentage of faculty from ethnic minorities will be roughly equivalent to the proportions of each group in the local population.

Table 12.3

Facilitative Strategies in Solving a Problem

1. Meet with faculty to discuss the concern, and foster ownership of the problem and of the desired outcome.
2. Investigate the resources in the community for identifying potential faculty members in the groups indicated.
3. Advertise in places targeted to the desired groups.
4. Work with a consultant to identify ways in which the environment is friendly or unfriendly to people in ethnic minorities.
5. Where problems are identified in #4, make appropriate changes.
6. Make prospective faculty members feel welcome and valued.
7. Openly share the concerns for a more ethnically diverse faculty group.
8. Once desired faculty are hired, make them feel welcome and facilitate their entry and retention within the system.

- external influences (such as the NLN);
- organizational structure;
- policies and procedures;
- power and influence patterns;
- resources (time, money, and people); and
- willingness to change of those involved.

During your planning, you must consider these factors and assess how each one fits in your situation as a constraint, an enabler, or both. Once you have made this assessment, you can determine how to surmount the constraints and how to activate the enablers. You should spend considerable time on this part of the process. If you overlook something, it may turn into a much more significant factor than you thought.

External influences would include accrediting bodies, such as the National League for Nursing or the regional accrediting body for your university. Other influences would be elements in the professional or local geographic community which may affect the change you are considering. In the case of the example shown in Tables 12.1-3, you would be concerned with the ethnic groups which you're interested in recruiting to your faculty.

Organizational structure is that structure within the school and the university which determines how decisions are made and enforced. If the desired change relates to the organization itself, your approach will need to take its structure into account. Being aware of this structure as it applies to the proposed change will help to facilitate the change.

Policies and procedures may determine how changes are implemented. For example, curriculum changes usually must be made through a specific committee or series of committees. Efforts to recruit and hire faculty are determined by policy. If you are trying to implement the proposed change regarding the ethnic makeup of the faculty, this will either have to be done according to the existing policies, or the policies themselves will need to be revised. For example, if your goal is to increase ethnic diversity, you cannot let faculty go who do not fit this description.

The lines of *power and influence* will affect your planning and implementation of any change. People with these attributes need to be recruited to support your proposal. They can use that power to help in moving along the process. If you ignore established powerful or influential faculty members, you are courting disaster.

Your *resources* of time, money, and people must be assessed. The more valued the proposed change and the wider your support, the more resources will be made available to help. However, in any school, there are still limits to these resources, no matter how dedicated the faculty are to a given change. For example, you may have qualified applicants who fit your criteria, but all of them live far from your campus. The expenses for interviewing all of them may be substantial. In deciding how to proceed, the dean and faculty must consider other priorities and determine if new allocations are feasible.

Some changes may require a different workload for faculty. You must decide whether this is realistic. For example, the faculty may want to offer some nursing courses more frequently in order to facilitate the way certain students move through the curriculum. This may mean that current faculty will have heavier loads, or that additional faculty will be required. You would need to determine whether either or both are possible given institutional resources.

Finally, the *willingness to change* must be assessed. If significant and influential people do not want the change, they may be able to squelch everyone else's efforts very quickly and effectively. Some other people may voice an interest in change, but may be consciously or unconsciously unwilling to participate. This can lead to serious problems if you do not thoroughly explore the willingness of the people involved. Situation 12.2 describes such an instance.

If you can accurately assess how willing your colleagues are to make a proposed change, you will be able to intervene to encourage them to be willing to change. If people are unwilling to change, you must find out what is at the root of this. There is always some motivation for any behavior. If you can discover this motivation, you will have the key to enlisting more support.

In some instances, people may be so miserable with a situation they are willing to make any change. This may cause problems, either because they are too willing to change and do so too rapidly, or because they do not investigate the possible consequences of

Unwillingness to Change

A group of faculty approached their dean to ask that efforts be made toward changing faculty attitudes and interest in using a specific model on which to base the curriculum. The faculty members felt this need was so obvious, that they did not assess the willingness of the dean to support such a change.

The dean was not really interested in undertaking a major curriculum revision which would be expensive in terms of faculty time, as well as having implications for other limited resources in the school. However, she felt she needed to placate the faculty who made the suggestion and look as if she were supporting a consideration of the possibility. She didn't want to antagonize those who wanted a change; she also didn't want to pressure those who were not convinced. Instead of finding a person well versed in nursing models who was also effective at communicating, she selected an uninspiring person who had only a minimal understanding of the principal nursing models herself. The resulting presentation had little effect on other faculty members' willingness to adopt a specific model. They felt justified in their decision, and the dean rationalized that she had tried to support the proposed change.

the change throughout the system. For example, faculty may decide to limit enrollment. If this is not well thought out and appropriately timed, there may be many disgruntled students and parents who had expected no difficulties in getting into nursing school. This can not only cause personal problems for the people directly affected, but also a feeling of ill will in the community at large.

CONCLUSION

Change is a process, whether it is planned or unplanned. To be most successful you must be able to clearly identify what needs to be changed and what the specific outcome will be that connotes success. Once you have thus defined your goal, you can work to use appropriate strategies to make the desired changes. Finally, any change has ethical implications which should be considered.

REFERENCES

Lewin, K. (1958). Group decision and social change. In T. M. Newcomb & E.L. Hartley (Eds.), *Readings in social psychology,* (3rd ed.). New York: Holt, Reinhart, & Winston.

Lippitt, G. (1973). *Visualizing change: Model building and the change process.* Fairfax, VA: NTL Learning Resources Corp.

Zaltman, G., & Duncan, R. (1977). *Strategies for planned change.* New York: Wiley.

THIRTEEN

Dealing with Disappointment

·······································

Academia is like the rest of life. Sometimes we don't get what we want, and sometimes very unpleasant things happen that may or may not be warranted by our own behavior. You must be realistic in anticipating disappointment. You also need to realize that you may be able to do little to change a bad situation. You must learn to anticipate situations in which there is a risk for you and plan for handling such situations.

PURPOSE

The purpose of this chapter is to help you to handle unpleasant events that are part of academia, and to learn to turn disappointments into opportunities.

SELF-CONCEPT AND SELF-ESTEEM

The most crucial things in helping you to deal with disappointment in any context are your self-concept and your self-esteem. The better you feel about yourself and your abilities, the more resilient you will be. Easily said, of course, but most of us have self-doubts, especially when we are new and inexperienced in a

173

situation. The key, over and over again, is to maintain the proper perspective.

To promote your self-esteem, you must determine what your value system is and learn how to function within it. The biggest threats posed to self-esteem are those things that challenge our values, and those times when we feel we haven't lived up to our own standards. When you're in a position to deal with your value system, you have to do so consciously or you'll be likely to disappoint yourself.

It is easy to feel that no one cares about you when you're feeling disappointed in yourself or feeling on the brink of or actually in burnout. These disappointments are part of a loss process, and the way to deal with them is cognitive: you have to work at thinking positive things about yourself and about others. This sounds so simple that I'm sure many people will overlook it or minimize its importance.

What keeps us feeling badly about ourselves or our lives is the way we *think* about those things. If we keep nurturing negative thoughts, we will be undermining ourselves all the time. However, if we replace those thoughts with positive ones, we shore up our self-esteem. I'm not saying you should ignore things that should be changed. Instead, you need to reframe them so that they will make you feel good about yourself.

For example, if you receive evaluations from students which indicate you're not doing as well as you want to, don't wallow in feeling sorry for yourself or in blaming the students. Look at what you can learn from them and formulate a plan for improving what needs to be improved. Then you can feel good about yourself for being willing and able to change. People who do not do this continue to carry around these negative perspectives, even if they appear as if they don't care what students think about them. Some teachers who consistently receive negative feedback from students never change and act as if it's only the students' problem. I can assure you that those people are not happy people, although they might appear to be. These negative experiences wear on people, they eventually pay for it, having a poorer quality of life than those who are willing to acknowledge their shortcomings and constructively work to change them.

EVALUATIONS

Evaluations are a part of life in academia. At times, you will be pleased, and feel they reflect your true skills as an educator. At other times, you will feel disappointed, unhappy, or even devastated by evaluations. Whether they are what you would like to hear or not, you need to consider evaluations as objectively as possible.

One reaction I have seen, especially in new people, is overreaction of faculty members to one or a few negative evaluations. All the others may be glowing with comments to back up whatever numerical scale is used, but those few that are negative will seem to outweigh all the others. This is a normal response, but you must learn to put the evaluations in perspective.

When you receive your evaluations, it's a good idea to ask someone more experienced to review them with you. You may want to choose another faculty member who has been teaching longer than you have to go over them with you and to help you adequately assess what they mean.

When you receive negative ratings or comments, consider what they might mean. One possibility is that what the students have said is absolutely correct. For example, the evaluation may report that you gave poor directions for an assignment. On reviewing these directions with you, your colleague and you may agree that they do need to be improved. This is the whole point of evaluations: to get feedback to help you to continue with your strong points or to improve your weak points.

At other times, the comments you receive may be vague and hostile and perplexing. For example, one of my students whom I had in clinical for community health once wrote that, "Ms. Schoolcraft never seemed to have time to listen to me. I didn't think she cared about how I was doing." This was mystifying to me, since I had met with each student for 15 minutes at the beginning of each clinical day, and for at least 15 minutes at the end, to review their plans and activities. This meant I met with most students at least an hour each week. In addition, I was available to talk with them at other times if the need arose. Since this particular student didn't elaborate, I couldn't really tell how I had failed her.

One reason the above example is illustrative is that the incident I described happened many years ago, but I still remember it. I still wonder what happened in my relationship with that student to make her feel that way and for her to make that comment. However, the way I dealt with this evaluation was just as I described: I analyzed the situation to see if I could account for how the problem could have happened, if it really did. Because I didn't know who the student was and couldn't figure out why any of them would feel that way, I couldn't correct whatever the problem was—if, indeed, there was really something I needed to correct.

This leads to a recognition of the overall factors about student evaluation of faculty that cause some of the discomfort. These factors include:

students are usually anonymous;

students may have unrealistic expectations of faculty; and

students may be vague about their comments or so general that the meaning is unclear.

BURNOUT IN ACADEMIA

Burnout is the disillusionment that follows "a confrontation with reality in which the human spirit is pitted against circumstances intractable to change" (Storlie, 1979, p. 2108). It is a common phenomenon that detracts from the personal and professional lives of many people. Fortunately, it is possible to design strategies to prevent burnout and its negative effects.

SIGNS OF BURNOUT

You can identify that you are in burnout when:

things that should be easy seem difficult;

things that should give you pleasure are neglected; and

you feel increasingly sad, disenchanted, cynical, and irritable.

These are the general characteristics, some more specific funny and not so funny signs are listed in Table 13.1.

ASSUMPTIONS

Several years ago, I conducted a series of workshops on burnout with a colleague, Clare Delaney. We developed eight assumptions

Table 13.1

Signs of Burnout

Moving family pictures back or covering them up on your desk.

Spending the first hours of each day attempting to figure out which project has the highest priority.

Making your highest priority tuning your radio so you can hear relaxing music.

Forgetting you have children.

Taking refuge in the elevator, copy room, or bathroom.

Stopping the elevator between floors and asking directions.

Beginning to believe your high school years really were the happiest days of your life.

Alphabetizing and filing your junk mail.

Waking up hours before the alarm goes off with a stomach ache or a headache on days you have to go to work.

Watching the clock.

Keeping your office door closed when you're there.

Feeling strong adverse feelings toward inanimate objects.

Experiencing constant *déja vu*.

Spending your time making lists of burnout symptoms.

Spending considerable amounts of time bitching about how others are not working as hard as you.

Leaving your home on a day off to go shopping and finding yourself pulling into the parking lot at work.

Cleaning out your filing cabinet rather than talking to students.

Thinking you're the only decent teacher on the faculty.

Becoming overly involved with students.

Becoming detached from students and other faculty.

From "Signs of Burnout," an unpublished manuscript by C. Delaney and V. Schoolcraft, 1980, Oklahoma City, OK: University of Oklahoma College of Nursing Continuing Education Program.

as a framework for designing strategies to cope effectively with or to prevent burnout. I will list these here as a possible guide to determine your own ways of dealing with burnout.

Assumption 1:

Suppressed feelings are often expressed in extreme behaviors, such as becoming totally detached or overly involved.

Assumption 2:

High idealism is virtually universal among nurses, and the clash of idealism with reality creates distress.

Assumption 3:

Human beings are capable of changing, but they may change or adapt in ways that are eventually dysfunctional for them.

Assumption 4:

Human beings are happier and more productive if meaningful work is adequately balanced with meaningful leisure activities.

Assumption 5:

Human beings are capable of learning throughout the life span.

Assumption 6:

Individuals can enhance their lives by meeting some needs through group involvement.

Assumption 7:

Individuals can contribute to their self-esteem by appreciating and acknowledging their own abilities and accomplishments.

Assumption 8:

The contribution of any individual may be limited by time, energy, and/or resources, regardless of that person's ability and motivation.

The purpose of delineating these assumptions is to help you to examine your own susceptibility to burnout as well as your capacity to deal with its onset. Although there may be others around you who will help you to deal with burnout, you are the best one to prevent it or cure it. Be aware of the warning signs mentioned earlier. If you detect them, review the above assumptions and consider how you might use them in treating your imminent burnout.

PREVENTIVE ACTIVITIES

The most significant factor in preventing or treating burnout is *intelligent self-interest*. If you think about all that has been said in the chapter about burnout signs and their related assumptions, you will have noted that one abiding characteristic of burnout is an overdeveloped sense that one's work is more important than oneself.

To restore your equilibrium, you need to do things that are in your self-interest. I added the modifier "intelligent" because it is important to use your head about manifesting self-interest. For example, one preventive is to take a break of some kind from your work. Simply abandoning your job, or taking a break that overburdens others, may not be smart because it will lead to other problems. By the same token, it is smart to make realistic assessments of the possibilities for such a break from work. Even though your absence may cause more work for some people, that does not mean that you don't deserve it or shouldn't take it.

Table 13.2 lists some activities to help in preventing burnout in general, as well as some which are specific to being an educator. You can initiate these activities for yourself as part of the intelligent self-interest I mentioned earlier.

Your administrators can also help to decrease stress and the resultant burnout. Some of these activities are listed in Table 13.3. Before you try to make any changes in response to these suggestions, investigate how many of them may already be possible. Read the school and university policies and talk with other faculty members to find out which of these are practical. Even if some are not a part of your institutional system you can make use of these suggestions by sharing them in a timely manner, either directly or indirectly, with your dean and others. You might be

Table 13.2

Preventing Burnout

Take care of yourself—physically, mentally, spiritually.

Develop interests outside of nursing and teaching.

Exercise control over your own life.

Listen to your own thoughts and feelings.

Maintain an inner sense of autonomy.

Develop a bond with other faculty in and out of nursing.

Recognize the place of ideals in the real world.

Seek new challenges.

Talk with colleagues about problems and feelings.

Continue to develop expertise in your area.

Take a break from work—a leave of absence, a summer off, or a sabbatical.

Reaffirm for yourself that what you're doing is right.

Team up with a colleague to teach a course.

Design a new course or revamp one you're already teaching.

From "Preventing Burnout," an unpublished manuscript by C. Delaney, 1980, Oklahoma City: OK-University of Oklahoma College of Nursing Continuing Education Program.

able to help formalize some of these through the appropriate school or university committees.

Frequently, when faculty members feel they're burning out, their deans or other associates are so busy themselves that they are unaware of the situation until it has progressed to an unhealthy stage. Remember that you are probably able to conceal some of your problems from others and that you have chosen to do so for good reasons. In addition, your colleagues are very busy. They can overlook your problems, but this need not mean that they're insensitive, or that they wouldn't be concerned if they knew of your difficulty.

Table 13.3

Organizational Preventives for Burnout

Reinforcing creativity and good teaching;

Decreasing paperwork;

Trusting faculty members;

Helping faculty to moderate contact with students who increase stress;

Providing rationale for organizational priorities and involving faculty in setting them;

Supporting faculty members to make changes;

Encouraging relationships between new faculty and experienced faculty members;

Planning for and supporting personal and professional development; and

Relieving faculty members of some responsibilities when they're feeling stressed.

MAJOR DISAPPOINTMENTS

Nothing in the following section is meant to discourage you from applying for a new position, advance in rank, or retention within the organization. If we live our whole lives only to avoid disappointment, we're doomed to a bland existence. However, we must approach such possibilities with realistic expectations of ourselves and others. Major disappointments would include such things as being rejected for a promotion in position or rank or being turned down for tenure or its equivalent.

PROMOTION

If you are vying with others for an advancement to a specific position, such as a course coordinator or assistant dean, you must meet the established criteria, but the grounds for choosing between you and others may be subjective. You must not only meet the standards of the institution, but you must also pay attention to the internal politics that will tell you what is going to influence the decision.

Frequently, when people are not advanced to certain positions, they have limited insight into the reasons. You will avoid disappointment if you are realistic about the organizational factors that contribute to such decisions. For example, if you don't already work well with the people you would be working with most in the prospective new situation, they're not likely to want you in it. Not only that, but you are probably better off not being in it.

ADVANCES IN RANK OR RETENTION

The most obvious way to avoid disappointments in being considered for advances in rank or in long-term retention is to understand the criteria for these achievements. To attain these advances, you must do the things necessary to meet the criteria. At best, you will receive the promotion in rank and/or tenure. At worst, if you clearly meet the criteria but do not receive the proper advance in rank or retention, you will have grounds for a grievance.

In some academic settings, there have been cases of faculty members who are advanced in rank or receive tenure without meeting the published criteria. This probably happens everywhere. If you happen to be the recipient of this sort of inequitable decision, you may feel it's a benefit, although you will be held in some degree of contempt by at least a few of your colleagues. If you are being considered for an advance in rank or for tenure, and even if you see that the criteria have been disregarded in the past, do not expect that they should be or will be suspended for you.

If you do not receive the advance or tenure and you clearly meet the criteria, you do have grounds for a grievance. This is the most appropriate response. However, such actions are time-consuming and emotionally draining. As with all disappointments, you must decide how much you are willing to do if you believe you have been treated unfairly. You have to weigh the risks and benefits to you and decide which things will determine your line of action. Once you have made a decision, you must have the courage to proceed.

If you decide to protest your treatment, you will find out who your true friends are. I can guarantee you that there are some people you thought you could always count on—people who vowed you could always count on them—who will turn against you. Others will not want to risk anything in their own situations to be seen as aligned with you. Therefore, in the spirit of intelligent self-interest, you need to nurture friendships with people who are courageous and who may be insulated from the risks that might discourage their support when you most need it.

At times, you may decide it is better to move on with your life than to protest the negative decision. The healthiest thing you can do is to look for ways in which to turn a disappointment into an opportunity. For example, if you don't receive the advance in rank, you probably don't have to leave the school. Instead take this as a "wake-up call" to become more productive. You may make such progress that you will find chances to do things you never knew existed. If you don't receive tenure and have to leave, do so gracefully. Consider the promise involved in being able to start fresh in a new situation. Get your professional life in order so that the next time you're considered, you won't be turned down.

The reality you must constantly confront in academia is that growth is expected. If you don't want to meet the established criteria within a given school or university, you must find a place where you can meet the criteria. Otherwise, you will never be able to settle into one place and stay there for an extended length of time. If you don't mind moving around in academia, you will be able to do so for a while in your career. However, you will eventually find it more and more difficult to get new positions, because as you age, you are also expected to grow professionally. If you don't have the credentials and accomplishments to show this growth, you'll have increasing difficulty in finding a faculty position.

If you look at almost any faculty group, you will probably see people who have "retired on the job," meaning they are still employed, but are not productive. What you will also see is that fewer people are getting the opportunity to do the same thing in each situation. Be good to yourself—and don't put yourself in the position of one of those people who has a minimal teaching load and is not respected by colleagues or students. Such a person may seem happy, but they do feel the ongoing contempt felt by others toward them. They may seem outwardly indifferent to these negative feelings, but they are paying the price emotionally for being neither respected nor respectable in the situation.

BEING COURAGEOUS IN ADVERSITY

Some of the disappointments we experience in academia are related to things that go on around us and that affect us even when they don't appear to directly. This includes circumstances pertaining to the leadership in the school or university. In most academic settings, faculty members have input into the appointments of major administrative officials. The nearer the administrator is to your position, the more input you are likely to have. However, the operative word here is *input*. By that I mean that you may have the opportunity to express your opinion, but those making the decision may disregard it completely.

When you do have the opportunity to give input, you should be as honest and open as possible without offering yourself as a sacrifice. You have to carefully assess the situation to see the risks you are taking by stating your opinion openly and honestly. If you choose not to be completely candid and open, you need to assess your own ability to live with that decision.

The truth is that it is sometimes so obvious that your opinion is irrelevant that you are better off not even sharing it. However, in some situations you will not be able to live with yourself if you don't take the risk to let others know what you think. When this is so, as the adage goes there is usually safety in numbers. If you feel very deeply that something unjust is happening, find out who else holds this concern. Even this may be dangerous, you may be opening yourself to risk by discussing the situation with the wrong people. Start with the people you feel you can trust the most. This is where all your political knowledge and skills will come into play. You have to figure out who is allied with whom, and avoid talking too openly with those who are your adversaries or with others whose allegiances are unclear. After some investigation, you will either have some compatriots, or you will know that you are alone. At that point, you must again decide if you're willing to take the risks inherent in making your beliefs known.

There are some situations in which you will take whatever risks you must to be true to your beliefs and values. Even though you may be courageous and handle yourself well, you may still not get the result you hope for.

CONCLUSION

In any academic setting, you will be faced with a certain amount of success and usually a certain number of disappointments. Some disappointments can be avoided with good planning and by following the guidelines suggested above. Others cannot be avoided but can be used to help you to grow. Some of the occasions which seem the most disappointing to you may actually be the best things to happen in your career.

REFERENCES

Delaney, C. (1980). Preventing burnout. Unpublished manuscript. Oklahoma City, OK: University of Oklahoma College of Nursing Continuing Education Program.

Delaney, C., & Schoolcraft, V. (1980). Signs of burnout. Unpublished manuscript. Oklahoma City, OK: University of Oklahoma College of Nursing Continuing Education Program.

Storlie, F. J. (1979). Burnout: The elaboration of a concept. *American Journal of Nursing, 79,* 2108–2111.

········**·FOURTEEN·**········

Becoming a Part of the Community of Scholars

●●●●●●●●●●●●●●●●●●●●●●●●●●●●●●●●●

The eventual result of all the processes described in this book is that you become a part of the community of scholars. This is one of those things you have to earn. It is rarely simply bestowed on anyone. You earn it by doing a good job and, to some extent, by doing what is expected of you.

The process includes learning the role that is expected of you. A part of this entails finding a mentor or guide who can help you as you develop your career. You must also work on your perspectives of reality inside your profession, as well as beyond it: into the rest of academia and into the community at large.

PURPOSES

The purposes of this chapter are to help you to:

- identify the importance of learning the role of scholar;
- find and work with a mentor or guide; and
- foster and maintain a broad-based view of academia.

LEARNING THE ROLE

Most of this book has described the typical things expected of faculty members in universities. You can easily learn what your responsibilities are. However, you may have more difficulty than you anticipate when you actually start trying to live in that role.

You can best cope with any disenchantment by starting out with as realistic a view as possible. If you have chosen teaching as your career because you think that teaching is all that teachers do, you are going to be very disillusioned. However, if you realistically consider all the aspects of the faculty role described in this book and elsewhere, you will be less likely to suffer enormous disappointment.

At first, most new faculty members are excited about being able to fulfill their dream to teach. They look at the course or courses in which they'll be teaching and feel a thrill at the thought of working with students. They think how well they will do emulating teachers they loved and avoiding the poor techniques of less appreciated teachers.

Then, reality sets in. Most of us find that, just as with most roles there are parts of this role that are drudge work. There are policies to be followed about preparing course materials; notices have to be issued to one person or another under certain circumstances; and other people and other factors infringe on your teaching time. You also discover that not every student is a willing or interested participant in your wonderful efforts.

You begin to realize just how much time is taken up by the ancillary responsibilities of a faculty member. Committee work and other quasi-administrative responsibilities demand a lot of your time. The expectation for you to do research and to write professionally at first seems challenging and welcome. However, as you begin to try to balance those expectations with your teaching load, the time for one may seem to be encroaching on the time for the other.

All of those feelings usually set in after the first year. In the first year of teaching, you will have fewer demands. However, after that, you will be expected to begin to fulfill more and more of the typical responsibilities that have been described throughout this book. To keep such feelings from discouraging you, you need to start with the right perspective. You must accept that all these activities are part of the role you want to take on. You must learn to handle the things you like least as gracefully as you do the things you like most. Fighting them or trying to avoid them will seldom make you happier and will usually bring you more, rather than fewer, headaches.

FINDING AND WORKING WITH A MENTOR

WHAT A MENTOR DOES

The definition I use of the mentor role is based on my research and the literature I reviewed in preparation for my dissertation. A *mentor* is an influential person who gives you significant help in reaching your major life goals. I call the person who is helped by a mentor a mentee. A mentor provides you with guidance and assistance in learning your role, actualizing your role attainment, and fulfilling your professional goals. The definition I use of the mentor role is based on my research and the literature I reviewed in preparation for my dissertation. Table 14.1 lists these components; they are discussed below as I have applied them to my own work with mentees.

The mentor—mentee dyad is a robust and comprehensive relationship between a novice and a more experienced professional person. I have served as a mentor for several colleagues. This is not something I can do with every promising student or colleague, because it takes a lot of time and energy to invest this effort. I have to be selective, and I need to see that my help will be valued and appreciated.

As a *teacher*, I help my mentees to learn factual information. This might be by simply telling them things I think they should know, or I might suggest reading or other activities for them. Often, I am or have been in a formal relationship with my mentees as their teacher, but my efforts extend beyond the limits of one course. In teaching them, I not only impart information, I also help them to learn *how* to learn throughout the rest of their careers.

In the aspect of a *sponsor*, I use my position and influence to help my mentees. If necessary, I help them to get into a professional position. I assist them in learning the ropes, so to speak, so that they can advance in their chosen area of practice. This is

Table 14.1

Roles of a Mentor

Teacher:

A mentor enhances the mentee's skills and intellectual development.

Sponsor:

The mentor uses influence to facilitate entry and advancement for the mentee.

Host and Guide:

The mentor welcomes the new initiate and acquaints the mentee with values, customs, resources, and people of concern.

Exemplar:

A mentor serves as a model.

Counselor:

A mentor provides advice and moral support in times of stress.

Realization of the Dream:

The mentor helps the mentee define the newly emerging self by supporting and facilitating the initiate's dream; the mentor believes in the mentee as a person and gives the mentee's dream her or his blessing.

most effective when the mentee has chosen to become an educator, since that is my current area of practice. However, I can be of some assistance even to those in clinical or administrative areas of practice.

As a *host and guide*, I see that my mentees become involved as professionals, regardless of their area of practice. I make sure they understand what is expected of a professional person. I help them to think about the image they project in terms of everything from their attire to the way they express themselves. I give them an idea of what to expect before they go to a meeting or other activity, and prepare them to behave in a professional manner. I see that they go to the right professional meetings, and while they're there, I make sure they meet people—other influential professionals, or perhaps people who are simply interesting. For example, I might introduce them to nursing theorists or to other nursing leaders whom they might feel shy about approaching alone. I make sure they know my friends and who they are.

Whenever possible, I get my mentees involved in organizational activities. I encourage them to volunteer for committee service in the district and state nurses association. I encourage them to be active in Sigma Theta Tau. If they have chosen a specialty organization with which to affiliate, I encourage them to be as active and interactive as possible with that group.

As an *exemplar* to my mentees, I try to serve as a model of professional behavior. I do not expect, nor do I need, my mentees to become clones of me. I appreciate their differing gifts. I merely provide them with a view of how I function as a professional. I try to be faithful to all the lessons I have given them about being an active member of organizations; about presenting myself professionally; and about speaking up and being well prepared when I do so.

I discuss my own activities with my mentees and help them to understand how I have chosen to do what I have done. I'm honest with them about my own concerns. For example, if I feel I haven't handled something well, I will share this with my mentees and let them help me analyze how I might have done things differently. One of the most valuable things we can do for those we want to help is to show them that we're not perfect either. We have misgivings and often wish we could have done better. On the other hand, I also share my ability to assess a situation and make effective decisions about proceeding.

I invite mentees to work with me on professional projects such as my research or writing. For example, I invited one of my mentees to co-author a chapter with me in an earlier book I edited. This man had a good knowledge base in the content involved, so he made a contribution in his own right. By working with me, he learned more about writing for publication and the process involved. It also gave him a special opportunity to get published. I worked with that same mentee in producing a presentation about men in nursing, which we delivered to several different audiences. Because of my experience and reputation, he was able to do this more easily than if he had tried it on his own or with an equally inexperienced colleague.

Sometimes I am a *counselor* for my mentees. Although this usually takes place in terms of their professional growth, I can also help them with other problems. I can give them assistance in figuring out solutions to personal problems when they feel overwhelmed. I have a background in mental health, so I am able to provide more counseling than someone without this background; but, if I think a mentee needs long-term or intensive counseling, I refer them to another professional. However, many of the stresses and strains which are normal in career development and personal growth can be discussed within the mentor-mentee relationship.

The ultimate service of the mentor is to help in the *realization of the dream* of the mentee. This means that I help each mentee to define herself or himself in a professional sense, and I convey my belief in their abilities to reach their goals. I do this by talking with them about their dreams. I make sure they know that I trust their judgment and respect their abilities. Inevitably, this means sending them on their own way.

FINDING A MENTOR

By seeing what I have done for mentees, you can get an idea of what a mentor might do for you. Levinson (1976, 1978) has done a great deal of research into the development of professional careers. He has described the relationship between a mentor and a mentee as a lot like falling in love. A certain "chemistry" is necessary to make the mentor want to give his or her time, and to attract the mentee to work with the mentor.

I like this analogy, because—just like falling in love—you can't simply will a relationship with a mentor or a mentee to happen. Just like romantic involvements, sometimes one party is more interested at first than the other. At other times, there seems to be an immediate mutual attraction. You can make yourself open to the experience and seek out a partner, but the relationship may or may not develop as you wish it would.

When you identify a prospective mentor, figure out for yourself why you want to work with that person. What abilities does that person have that attract you? Is the person an accomplished researcher, a master teacher, or an expert clinician? An easy first step is to let the prospective mentor know that you're interested in her or his work. Talk to the person about her or his research, teaching, or clinical practice. Talk about your own goals and related interests. If there's something specific you want to learn, ask about it.

If the person is doing research, volunteer to help. Almost any researcher can use an assistant to help distribute materials, track down references, or tabulate data. If the prospective mentor is a teacher, enroll for a class or ask to take a directed reading with her or him. If the person is a clinician, find a way to work in their clinical area. This gives you the chance to show what you are like and to interest the other person in working with you.

There's also nothing wrong with simply asking for such a relationship. Tell the prospective mentor what you think they have to offer and why you would like to work more closely with them. Explain what you hope to get out of the relationship and what you expect to put into it. Be aware that your prospective mentor may not necessarily be interested. She or he may want someone more educationally advanced or someone with more research skills. Not everyone wants to be a mentor, or people who may be interested may not be available at the time you want them to be.

Sometimes, a mentor will pick you. This has always been the case with me. I have had three mentors. None of these relationships started out as a conscious decision. They simply evolved, and it was only in retrospect that I realized they filled the description.

As a mentor, I have either selected my mentees, or a mutual attraction has grown into that kind of relationship. Most of my mentees have first been my students, but a few have been younger colleagues.

Just as in romantic attachments, you will sometimes be disappointed. You may find out that your mentor cannot provide the degree of help you want and need. Your mentor may lose interest in you or have to devote more attention to her or his own career or problems. Your mentor may be more involved with other mentees than with you. Although any of these eventualities may be painful, you need to put them into perspective and avoid discouragement. Move on and look for another person who can help you.

On the other hand, mentor–mentee relationships often grow into something else. Some become a close and long-lasting friendship, rather than a strictly professional relationship. I am still in contact with all of the people I have considered to be my mentors, as well as with those I have mentored. My mentors care about my continued growth, and I know I can still contact them for some of the same reasons as when I was a less experienced professional. By the same token, some of my mentees are still in active relationships with me, while others have only occasional contact to keep me abreast of what is going on in their lives. I have had the honor of becoming close enough to one that she asked me to be the godmother of her daughter. Another did me the honor of naming a cat after me. (Since I love cats, this may have meant more to me than it would to some people.)

A BROAD-BASED VIEW OF THE COMMUNITY OF SCHOLARS

One thing I have found to be common among many of my colleagues is that they have too narrow a view of academia and their place in it. They have become so focused on their own little corner of the world that they misperceive the relative importance of what is going on there.

STAR TREATMENT

Most of us have to follow all the rules, such as serving on committees, publishing a certain amount, and doing student advisement. Not all of us like all of these aspects of the role, but we have to fulfill them to stay in the university and to advance. It is only the occasional "star" who can bypass parts of the role. This is one part of reality you need to know about and simply accept. Don't waste your energy complaining if someone else doesn't seem bound by these rules.

One of my friends was on the same faculty as a Nobel Prize winner. She said he never participated in committees, and pretty much did as he pleased. He still advanced in rank and got tenure, although he didn't put much effort into fulfilling or documenting the respective criteria. Many other faculty members groused about this behavior, to no avail. The bottom line is that the presence of such a person on your faculty is an enormous benefit to the university, and such people will nearly always get special treatment in order to keep them there. My advice is to try to accept this fact of life, put it in perspective, and go on with what you need to do.

NURSING EDUCATION

There are some ways in which all schools of nursing are very similar. However, there are many more ways in which they are all quite different. Even though the structure may be similar from one to another, each school and its larger institution has evolved in its own way. You should try to learn how other schools and universities operate. Talk to colleagues at professional meetings, or read professional journals. Your goal is not to be able to describe all the different schools, but to gain an appreciation of their many differences.

To be an effective educator, you need to have a sense of the past as well as the present of nursing education. If you want to change anything—from the way you make assignments to the entire curriculum—you must know something of how these things have evolved in nursing education. This will keep you from making mistakes, and will enhance your successes.

You must know about the organizations which have an impact on higher education and nursing education. You need a sense of how change occurs in academia. Even if you have classes which touch on these issues, you will still have plenty to learn when you graduate. To be an effective and responsible faculty member, you need to be aware of what is going on in nursing education all over the country, and especially in your own vicinity.

THE NURSING PROFESSION

You must be knowledgeable about what is happening within your own profession. Stay current on the issues not only within your local vicinity and the state, but within the region, nationally, and internationally. This is relatively easy to do through such publications as *The American Nurse, The American Journal of Nursing, Nurs-*

ing Outlook, Nursing and Health Care, Image and many other journals. You should subscribe to at least one or two. In addition, you can go to your school library and look at the tables of contents of the current periodicals. I regularly circulate photocopies of the tables of contents of the journals I receive to my colleagues on the faculty. If they see a topic that looks interesting, they can borrow the journal. Another faculty member does something similar for all the journals which contain mostly research articles.

Attend local and state nursing meetings on a regular basis. You can learn a lot from such activities, not only in formal meetings but through the informal interactions you have there. When you go to meetings, make it a point to meet and talk to people from places other than your own school. When you attend a luncheon or dinner, try to arrange to sit with people you don't see often, and really talk to them about what's going on where they are. If possible, attend national meetings. Spend time with new people as well as old friends. I enjoy traveling to such meetings with friends, but I always try to spend some time meeting new folks. This is an excellent experience, and I learn a lot from my new acquaintances.

Get active as a committee member or officer within your district or state nurses association. This is not only good experience, it is a good way to stay well informed. You have the opportunity to meet and work with a wider variety of nurses than those you see every day. This involvement keeps you in touch with the concerns of other nurses, not just those where you take your students for clinical experience.

Talk to your dean and other senior colleagues about what's happening in the profession. You will find that they may have different perspectives and opinions about the same events. This will help you to consider your own ideas.

ACADEMIA

In addition to being well informed about your own profession and nursing education, you need to have a wide perspective on higher education. You should read at least one publication regularly which keeps abreast of higher education on a national level. The best resource for this is *The Chronicle of Higher Education,* which reports events on campuses all over the country and also helps to put them into a perspective which can help even the novice faculty member to appreciate the issues involved.

You must venture into the rest of the university and not restrict yourself to the school of nursing. Volunteer for committee assignments and other activities which will give you the opportunity to meet your colleagues in other fields. Talk with faculty in other disciplines about the issues which concern you. You will gain a wealth of information from the points of view of faculty members who may teach much differently than you. You will also find much common ground for sharing your concerns and ideas.

WIDER PERSPECTIVES

You must be aware of the trends and resources which affect higher education. Read the newspapers and watch the news for stories which have an impact on education, such as changes in elected officials and budgeting for education. Private as well as public institutions are affected by state and national politics and the economy.

To be a fully contributing member of academia, you must take some interest in state and national politics. Even if all you feel you can do is to vote, at least do that. However, you may feel you can do more: help in candidates' campaigns, write letters to your representatives, or serve as an advisor on nursing and health care to a representative. All of these activities will add to your knowledge and influence as well as perform a real service for the community.

CONCLUSION

Becoming a part of the community of scholars is a career-long task. It is more than arriving at a destination; it is a way of proceeding with your career. You spend the first part of your career learning your role and finding others to help you to confirm it. Then you spend the rest of your life in academia living the role and helping newer colleagues to learn as you did. You must know what you want and be well aware of the community around you as it expands around you in ever-widening circles. To be a part of the community of scholars is to make a commitment to yourself and to others to continue to grow throughout your career, and to always do your best for the students and others whose lives you touch.

REFERENCES

Levinson, D.J., Darrow, C.N., Klein, E.B., Levinson, M.H., & McKee, B. (1976). Periods in the devewlopment of men: Ages 18 to 45. *The Counseling Psychologist, 6,* 21–25.

Levinson, D.J., Darrow, L.N., Klein, E.B., Levinson, M.H., & McKee, B. (1978). *The seasons of a man's life.* New York: Ballantine.

Sample Curriculum Vitae

·····························

Mary C. Lowe   SS# 012−34−5678
1010 N. Woods Dr.   U.S. Citizen
Miami Groves, FL 33130   FL RN license #00012345
(405) 555−1234   MO RN license #99988123

EDUCATION

1986	Ph.D., Walker University, Miami Groves, FL, Nursing Science
1979	M.S.N., Henderson University, Kansas City, MO, Nursing Education
1974	B.S.N., Lavinia Dock School of Nursing, Henderson University, Kansas City, MO

PROFESSIONAL EXPERIENCE

1989−Present	Associate Professor, College of Nursing, Walker University, Miami Groves, FL
1986−1989	Assistant Professor, College of Nursing, Walker University
1982−1986	Instructor, College of Nursing, Walker University
1979−1982	Instructor, Lavinia Dock School of Nursing, Henderson University, Kansas City, MO
1977−1979	Assistant Head Nurse, Pediatric Nursing Unit Community Hospital, Kansas City, MO

1974–1977   Staff Nurse, Pediatric Nursing Unit,
Community Hospital, Kansas City, MO

AWARDS AND HONORS

1991   Outstanding Faculty Member of the Year,
College of Nursing, Walker University

1991   Professional Achievement Award, Walker University

1986   Phi Delta Kappa, National Honor Society in
Education, inducted into Zeta Omicron Chapter

1986   Outstanding Dissertation Award, College of
Education, Walker University

1985   Excellence in Writing Award, Florida Nurses
Association

1974   Sigma Theta Tau, International Honor Society for
Nursing, inducted into Zeta Alpha Chapter

PUBLICATIONS

Lowe, M. C. (1991). When a child dies. *Oncology Nurse, 4*, 120–124.

Lowe, M. C. (1990). Responses of novice nurses to the death of a child. *Research in Pediatric Oncology, 19*, 211–213.

Lowe, M. C. (1988). Coping mechanisms in pediatric oncology nurses. *Research in Pediatric Oncology, 17*, 71–73.

Lowe, M. C. (1982). The child with cancer. In J. S. Duncan (ed.), *Pediatric nursing,* pp. 276–291. New York: Bartley.

Lowe, M. C. & Carson, L. D. (1986). Why nurses belong to their state nurses association. *Professional Association, 25,* 72–76.

RESEARCH

Preparation of parents with terminally ill children (data collection in progress)

Responses of novice nurses to the death of a child, 1988–1989 (Funded in part by Zeta Zeta Chapter of Sigma Theta Tau)

Coping mechanisms in pediatric oncology nurses, doctoral dissertation, 1986

Lecture vs. seminar as a teaching method for undergraduate nursing students, masters thesis, 1979

INSTITUTIONAL SERVICE

1990–1992	Pediatric Department Coordinator, School of Nursing
1987–1992	Curriculum Committee, School of Nursing
1990–1992	Grants and Awards Committee, University
1983–1987	Student Affairs Committee, School of Nursing
1980–1982	Curriculum Committee, College of Nursing

PROFESSIONAL MEMBERSHIPS

1988–Present	Florida League for Nursing/NLN
1984–Present	Florida Association of Pediatric Nurses
1983–Present	Oncology Nurses Association
1982–Present	Florida Nurses Association/ANA
	District Program Committee (1988–1990; 1990–1992, Chair)
	Delegate to FNA House (1988, 1989, 1991, 1992)
	State Bylaws Committee (1991–1993)
1982–Present	American Educational Research Association
1974–1982	Missouri Nurses Association/ANA
1974–Present	Sigma Theta Tau International Honor Society of Nursing
	Zeta Zeta Chapter (1982–Present): Program Committee (1986–1988)
	Zeta Alpha Chapter (1974–1982): Program Committee (1978–1982)

PROFESSIONAL MEETINGS

1992	Florida League for Nursing Convention
1992	American Nurses Association Convention, Las Vegas, NV
1991	Sigma Theta Tau International Convention, Tampa, FL
1984,1991	Oncology Nurses Association Symposia
1984–1992	Florida Nurses Association Conventions
1979–1982	Missouri Nurses Association Conventions

CONTINUING EDUCATION PRESENTED

1992   Getting Your Research Published, Zeta Zeta Chapter Research Day

1991   Oncology Nursing with Children, Oncology Nurses Association Symposium, West Palm Beach, FL

1990   Care of Families with Terminally Ill Children, District Nurses Association, Miami, FL

1990   Planning Better Programs, FNA Convention, Marco Island, FL

1989   Talking to Children about Death, FNA Convention, Orlando, FL

1988   Responses of Novice Nurses to the Death of a Child, Zeta Zeta Chapter Research Day

CONTINUING EDUCATION ATTENDED

1992   Zeta Zeta Chapter Research Day, Miami Groves, FL (6 CEUs)

Nursing Theorist Conference, Baptist Medical Center, Miami, FL (12 CEUs)

Oncology Nurses Association Symposium, West Palm Beach, FL (8 CEUs)

Nursing: Shaping the Future of Health Care, FNA Convention, Ft. Lauderdale, FL (1 CEU)

The Ethics of Writing and Publishing, FNA Convention, Ft. Lauderdale, FL (1 CEU)

1991   Zeta Zeta Chapter Research Day, Miami, FL (6 CEUs)

Nursing Theorist Conference, Cedars Medical Center, Miami, FL (14 CEUs)

Nurses Care for America: Past and Present, FNA Convention, Jacksonville, FL (1 CEU)

Florence Nightingale portrayal, FNA Convention, Jacksonville, FL (1 CEU)

Mentorship: Cultivating the Future, FNA Convention, Jacksonville, FL (1.5 CEUs)

Reflections of Caring, Coping, and Commitment, Council on Child Health, FNA Convention (1 CEU)

Sigma Theta Tau International, Scientific, Program, & Leadership Sessions, Tampa, FL (19.6 CEUs)

1990   Negotiating for Care, FNA Convention, Marco Island (2 CEUs)

Building Teamwork Between Professional Tribes, FNA Convention (2 CEUs)

Humor and Caring, FNA Convention (1 CEU) Conference on Clinical Excellence in Nursing, Lambda Chi Chapter, Sigma Theta Tau (4 CEUs)

Dynamics of Developing Resources, Sigma Theta Tau Regional Assembly, Atlanta, GA (7.5 CEUs)

COMMUNITY SERVICE

1992	Red Cross volunteer, at Homestead Hurricane Relief Center
1989–1992	Volunteer group counselor, bereavement group, South Miami Hospital
1991	Volunteer to help immunize Haitian immigrants
1987–1989	Board member for Miami Groves Children's Mental Health Association
1984–1990	Volunteer in adult literacy education

Index

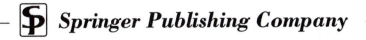
Springer Publishing Company

THE NURSE EDUCATOR IN ACADEMIA
Strategies for Success

Theresa M. Valiga, RN, EdD
and **Helen J. Streubert**, RN, EdD
Foreword by **Patricia Moccia**, PhD, RN, FAAN

"This is a wonderful book for anyone experiencing academia for the first time. Divided into five units, it can easily be read in its entirety or used as a stand-alone reference in relation to specific faculty roles or issues. ...a book to be shared during orientation of new faculty on any campus."
—American Journal of Nursing

Contents:

I: Entering and Understanding the Academic System. Letters. The First Faculty Appointment • The Academic Unit in Nursing: Key Players and Influential Strategies • Nursing as an Integral Part of the Academic Community • The National League for Nursing: Ally or Adversary?

II: Thriving in Academe. Letters. Faculty Work Load: What It Entails and Getting It All Done • Promotion and Tenure

III: Providing Quality Education. Letters. Implementing the Curriculum Model: Negotiating Student Learning Experiences • Education and Service: Interdependent Players in Nursing • Evaluation of Students: A Major Faculty Responsibility

IV: **Student-Related Issues for Faculty Members. Letters.** Traditional and Diverse Learners in Nursing: Admission, Progression, and Maintenance of Standards • The Failing Student: The Trials of Fulfilling One's Responsibility • The Teacher's Responsibility for Protecting the Rights of Students and Patients

V: Faculty Evaluation. Letters. The "Who," "What," "Where," "Why," and "How" of Faculty Evaluation • Faculty Evaluation as a Tool for Professional Growth

Springer Series on the Teaching of Nursing
1991   240pp   0-8261-7150-8   hardcover

536 Broadway, New York, NY 10012-3955 • (212) 431-4370 • Fax (212) 941-7842

Springer Publishing Company

AN ADDICTIONS CURRICULUM
For Nurses and Other Helping Professionals:
Volumes I and II

Elizabeth M. Burns, RN, PhD, FAAN,
Arlene Thompson, RN, PhD, and
Janet K. Ciccone, MA, APR, Editors

These two volumes present a comprehensive model program for teaching nurses about alcohol and drug addiction. It is specifically designed to be integrated into existing nursing courses, but can also be taught as a separate course. Both classroom and hands-on clinical learning are covered. Volume I is designed for undergraduates and includes a special section on training faculty. Volume II is for graduate and advanced-level students.

Volume I: Basic Knowledge and Practice
Contents: Foreword, *H. Werley* • Guide to Using The Addicitons Curriculum • Introduction to Alcohol and Other Drug Use, Abuse, and Dependence: A Focus on Education and Prevention, *A. Thompson* • The Psychosocial Effects of Chemical Abuse and Dependence, *C. Bininger* • Chemical Dependence: Assessment and Prevention of Medical Complications, *C.A. Baker* • Clinical Experiences with Treatment of Chemical Dependence (Tertiary Dependence), *A. Thompson and C. Bininger* • Professional, Legal, and Ethical Issues: An Integrative Seminar, *C. Bininger and A. Thompson* • Faculty and Staff Development: Chemical Dependence and Nursing Education, *A. Thompson & B. Melragon*

288pp   0-8261-8190-2   softcover

Volume II: Advanced Knowledge and Practice
Contents: Foreword, *H. Werley* • Introduction: Concept and Content • Health Promotion and Risk Reduction for Use and Misuse of Alcohol and Other Psychoactive Drugs, *M. E. Wewers* • Central Nervous System Effects of Psychoactive Drugs, *E.M. Burns and J.D. Wagner* • Chemical Dependence Issues of School-Age Youth and Adolescents, *E.M. Menke* • Interventions with Families Experiencing Chemical Dependence, *J.A. Clement* • Older Adults and Alcohol, Psychoactive Drugs, and Over-the-Counter Drugs: Misuse, Abuse, and Dependence, *J.S. Stevenson* • Central Nervous System Effects of Psychoactive Drugs: A Review, *E.M. Burns*

1993   392pp   0-8261-8191-0   softcover

536 Broadway, New York, NY 10012-3955 • (212) 431-4370 • Fax (212) 941-7842

Springer Publishing Company

A NUTS AND BOLTS APPROACH TO TEACHING NURSING

Victoria Schoolcraft, RN, MS, PhD

"A survival manual for those who are teaching for a brief time, for those who will eventually work on expanding their knowledge through formal coursework, or for those who are new at teaching and need a reference book. It is also intended to be a refresher for teachers who may not have done some of these things for a while."

—From the Preface

Contents:

Making Clinical Assignments • Supervising a Clinical Group • Designing a Learning Contract • Teaching Students to Work in Groups • Planning and Giving a Lecture • Planning and Facilitating a Seminar • Designing and Implementing a Course • Selecting Textbooks and Reading Assignments • Designing and Grading a Major Assignment • Designing and Grading a Minor Assignment • Constructing and Analyzing a Test • Facilitating Student Use of Computers • Guiding Independent Study • Helping Students to Improve Writing Skills

Springer Series on the Teaching of Nursing
Nurse's Book Society Selection
1989   224pp   0-8261-6600-8   *hardcover*

536 Broadway, New York, NY 10012-3955 • (212) 431-4370 • Fax (212) 941-7842

Springer Publishing Company

THEORY-DIRECTED NURSING PRACTICE

Shirley M. Ziegler, PhD, RN, Editor

The book first describes and then illustrates the use of critical thinking in moving from theory to the actual steps of the nursing process. Client cases are presented, and competing theories that might be used to direct nursing process are briefly introduced. Finally, one theory is selected for illustration for each case. The volume covers a range of theorists not found in other texts, including Aguilera, Messick, Bandura, Beck, Bowen, Erickson, Lazarus, Lewin, and Thomas.

Contents:

1993   280pp   0-8261-7630-5   hardcover

536 Broadway, New York, NY 10012-3955 • (212) 431-4370 • Fax (212) 941-7842